AN ARTIST'S PERSPECTIVE ON THE EYE

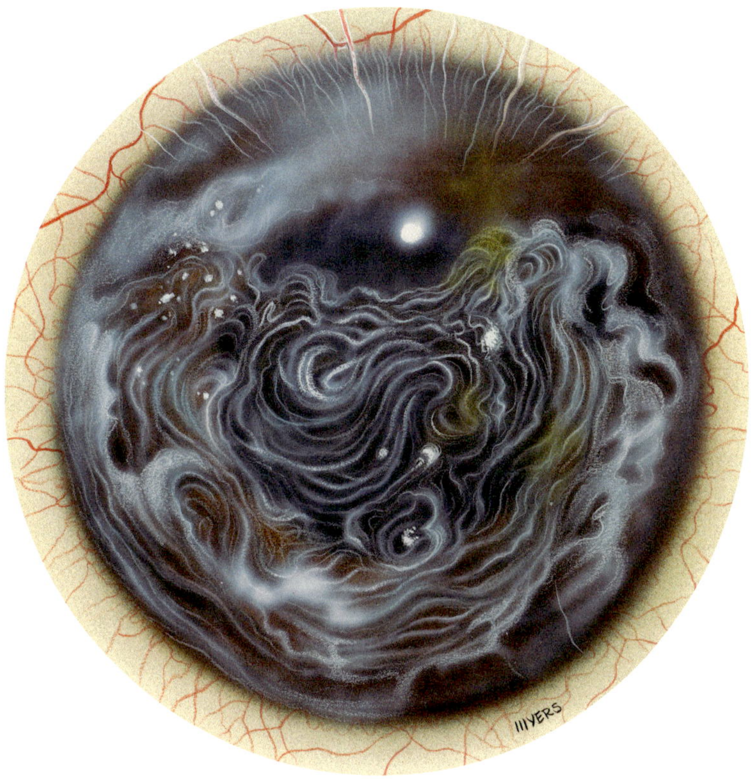

PAINTINGS BY J. McGUINNESS MYERS

An Artist's Perspective on the Eye - Paintings by J. McGuinness Myers

Published by the Bascom Palmer Eye Institute in cooperation with Fine Arts Press

This first edition of "An Artist's Perspective on the Eye - Paintings by J. McGuinness Myers" is comprised of 2,000 copies which includes a limited, numbered edition of 500 copies with slipcase.

This publication is typeset in Bodoni Antiqua, Garamond Regular and Bold.

Catalogue designed by Ron Shore, Shore Design, California
Photography by Richard Stratton
Publication coordinated by Richard K. Forster, MD
Edited by Reva Hurtes

ISBN: 978-0-9819933-6-2

Distributed by Fine Arts Press
www.fineartspress.com

Printed in Hong Kong

Cover illustration:
Coats Disease
[see also plate 78]

Frontispiece illustration:
Reis-Bücklers Corneal Dystrophy
[see also plate 10]

Title page illustration:
Coats Disease
[see also plate 78]

Foreword illustration, page 10:
Christmas Tree Cataract
[see also plate 48]

AN ARTIST'S PERSPECTIVE ON THE EYE

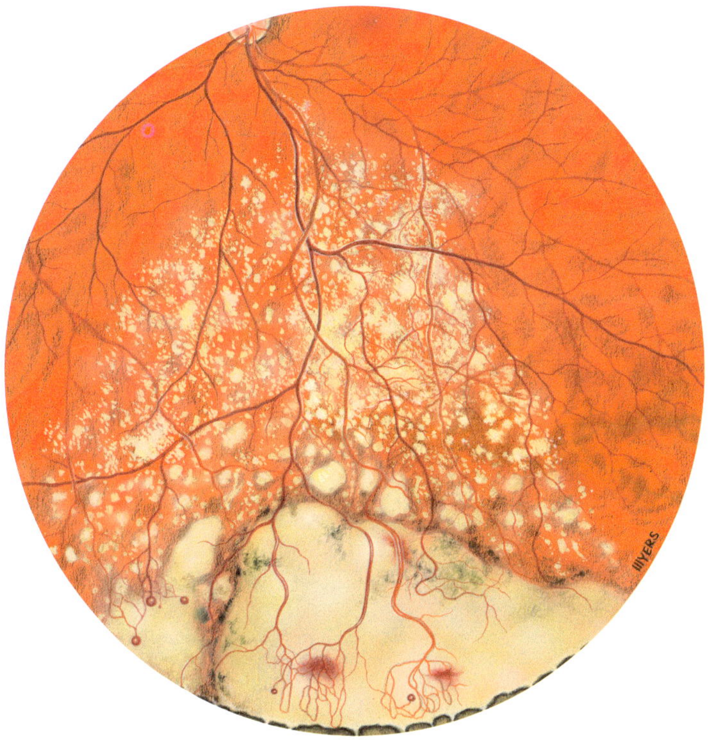

PAINTINGS BY J. McGUINNESS MYERS

Richard K. Forster, MD

Foreword by Helen L. Kohen with contributions by Andrew A. Moshfeghi, MD, MBA

Bascom Palmer Eye Institute

Department of Ophthalmology, University of Miami Miller School of Medicine

ACKNOWLEDGMENTS

We gratefully acknowledge the following individuals who have made significant contributions to this publication:

Helen L. Kohen, former Art Critic of the Miami Herald, for writing the Foreword

Bernice Steinbaum, of the Bernice Steinbaum Gallery in Miami, for her advice and suggestions

Ron Shore of Shore Design for the design, production and printing of this publication

Richard Stratton and his colleagues in the Photography Department of the Bascom Palmer Eye Institute, for their contributions and assistance including: Brenda Fallas, Giselle De Oliveira, Bridget Priedel, Alexander Rodriguez, Jennifer Thomson, MFA, Andrea Wildner, CRA, and Ditte J. Hess, CRA

Andrew A. Moshfeghi, MD, MBA, Associate Professor of Ophthalmology, Bascom Palmer Eye Institue, for contributing to the retinal paintings descriptions

Reva Hurtes, former Library Director at Bascom Palmer Eye Institute, for editing the text

Doris Silver, former Archivist at Bascom Palmer Eye Institute, for writing the original history on Mr. Myers

Cynthia Birch, Director of the Norton Library and Health Information Center and Dennis Bermudez, Senior Staff Assistant, for their assistance in providing access to the paintings and many helpful suggestions

The family of James C. Major, MD, for lending the paintings and giving permission to digitalize and publish the art in their possession (Plates 12 to 16, 19 to 22, 25 to 28 and 31)

Mrs. J. Donald M. Gass and family, for lending the three paintings (Plates 59, 60 and 61) and permission to digitalize and publish them

John Soucy, Director of Development and Ileana Daly-Bronstein, Director of Major Gifts, Development Department, Bascom Palmer Eye Institute

Eduardo C. Alfonso, MD, Professor and Chairman, Department of Ophthalmology, Director, Bascom Palmer Eye Institute

Michael Gittelman, Executive Director of the Anne Bates Leach Eye Hospital/Bascom Palmer Eye Institute

This publication would not be possible without the financial support and philanthropy of some very special patients and friends of the Bascom Palmer Eye Institute:

Ana and Guido Adler, for a major gift and personal support of this project

Marcella Werblow, a second generation donor to the Bascom Palmer Institute, and for introducing us to Helen L. Kohen

Steve Charles, MD, former resident at BPEI , who had the opportunity to know Mr. Myers while he was a medical student at the University of Miami School of Medicine

Mrs. Maria Tanska-Mills

Sylvan A. Schotz, MD

Dr. Richard K. and Janet F. Forster

TABLE OF CONTENTS

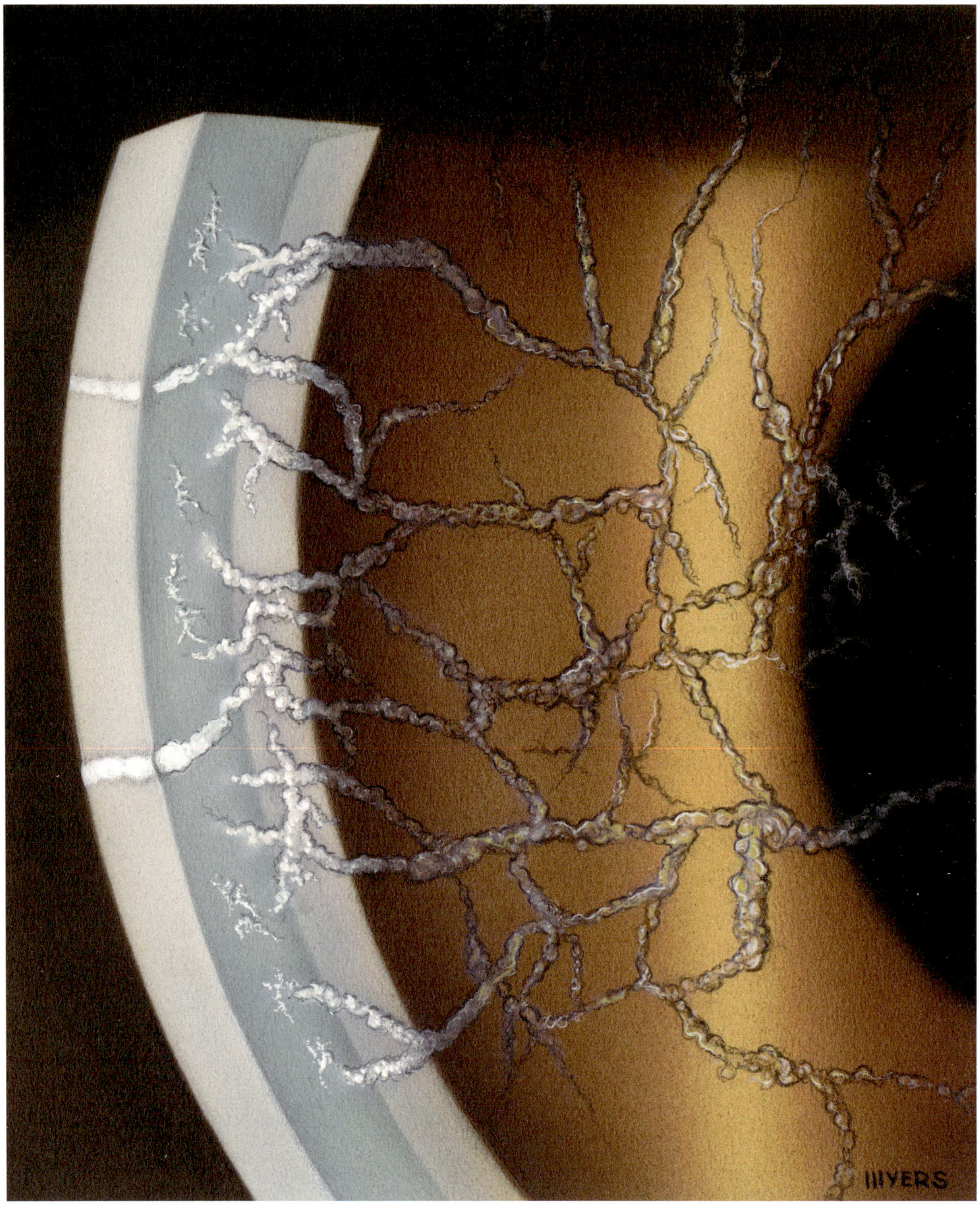

Fig. 1.

INTRODUCTION

RICHARD K. FORSTER, MD

It is a privilege for me to help facilitate and contribute to the publication of "An Artist's Perspective on the Eye—Paintings by J. McGuinness Myers." It is also especially appropriate to honor Mr. Myers in 2012, as the Bascom Palmer Eye Institute celebrates its 50th anniversary. In 1966, J. McGuinness Myers was hired by Dr. Edward W. D. Norton, founder of the Bascom Palmer Eye Institute and Chairman of the Department of Ophthalmology at the University of Miami School of Medicine. To quote the historical notes from the archives of the Mary and Edward Norton library:

> "J. McGuinness Myers, a medical illustrator who at one time lived in Ridgefield, Connecticut, was retired and living in Ft. Lauderdale, Florida when he accepted a job at BPEI in 1966. He remained at the Institute until his untimely death in 1968. Examples of his early work can be found in the two volume edition of *Biomicroscopy of the Eye, Slit Lamp Microscopy of the Living Eye* by M. L. Berliner, MD. Mr. Myers' personal copies can be found in the Rare Book Room of the Mary and Edward Norton Library of Ophthalmology.
>
> Volume I (1943) has 512 illustrations including 40 pages of color plates. The Preface to the volume contains the following reference to Mr. Myers: *I wish to thank especially Mr. J. McGuinness Myers for the long and tedious hours spent in making the illustrations....* Also in the front of the book is a handwritten inscription from the author dated 10/6/43 which reads: *To J. McGuinness Myers—Here it is! Again allow me to express my gratitude. We both shall remember the travail and horror of it all. But now on with the next. M.L.B.* Volume II (1949) of *Biomicroscopy of the Eye* has 1233 illustrations including 503 in color and is inscribed: *To Jack—to my partner in crime—the poor author M. L. Berliner.*"
>
> Mrs. Myers, Louise Wallingford Myers, was an illustrator for children's books including Golden Books, Random House.

Myers was able to uniquely capture and beautifully illustrate in these paintings on paper mounted on board what Henry David Thoreau described as "The noblest feature, the eye, is the fairest-colored, the jewel of the body." The purpose of this publication is therefore, to showcase the complete works of J. McGuinness Meyers during his all-too brief time at the BPEI. During the abbreviated three years, the first paintings of amyloidosis of the vitreous were completed in May, 1966 (Plates 51–58), and more than 100 paintings were completed by December, 1967—during about 20 months. Apparently, only two paintings were completed in 1968 shortly before his final illness: in January (Plate 81) and one in black and white in August (Plate 86). This ophthalmic art was not meant to be a comprehensive compilation of eye diseases and conditions, as were his paintings in Berliner's two volume text, but rather to illustrate specific conditions that might lend themselves to artistic illustration as the patients presented to the full-time faculty and community ophthalmologists, and physicians in training at the BPEI.

In addition, at the time although retinal photography was well developed and one-dimensional photographs of the cornea and anterior portions of the eye were taken with the Donaldson stereo camera, three-dimensional slit photography had not been well developed. Therefore, as one peruses the paintings in this book, many of the corneal illustrations include a three-dimensional slit-view (Fig. 1) with some only as a slit-view, that allows for appreciation of the depth of the lesions (Plates 9, and 37 to 41). Thus, through this technique, a detailed dimension was added that could not be illustrated by then current photography.

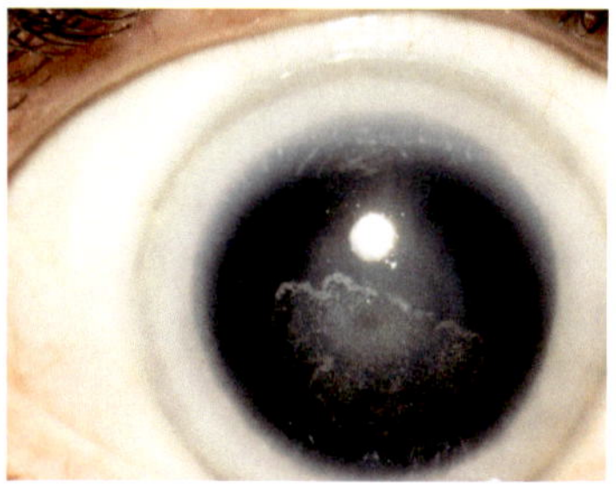

Fig. 2a.

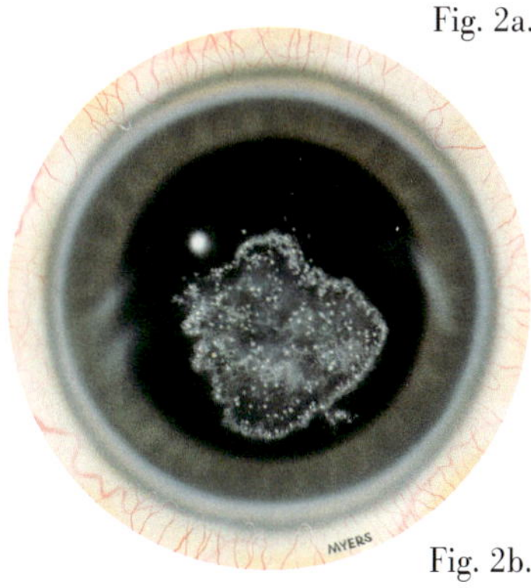

Fig. 2b.

The techniques used by Myers to arrive at a completed painting, included photos of the condition (Fig. 2a), sketches

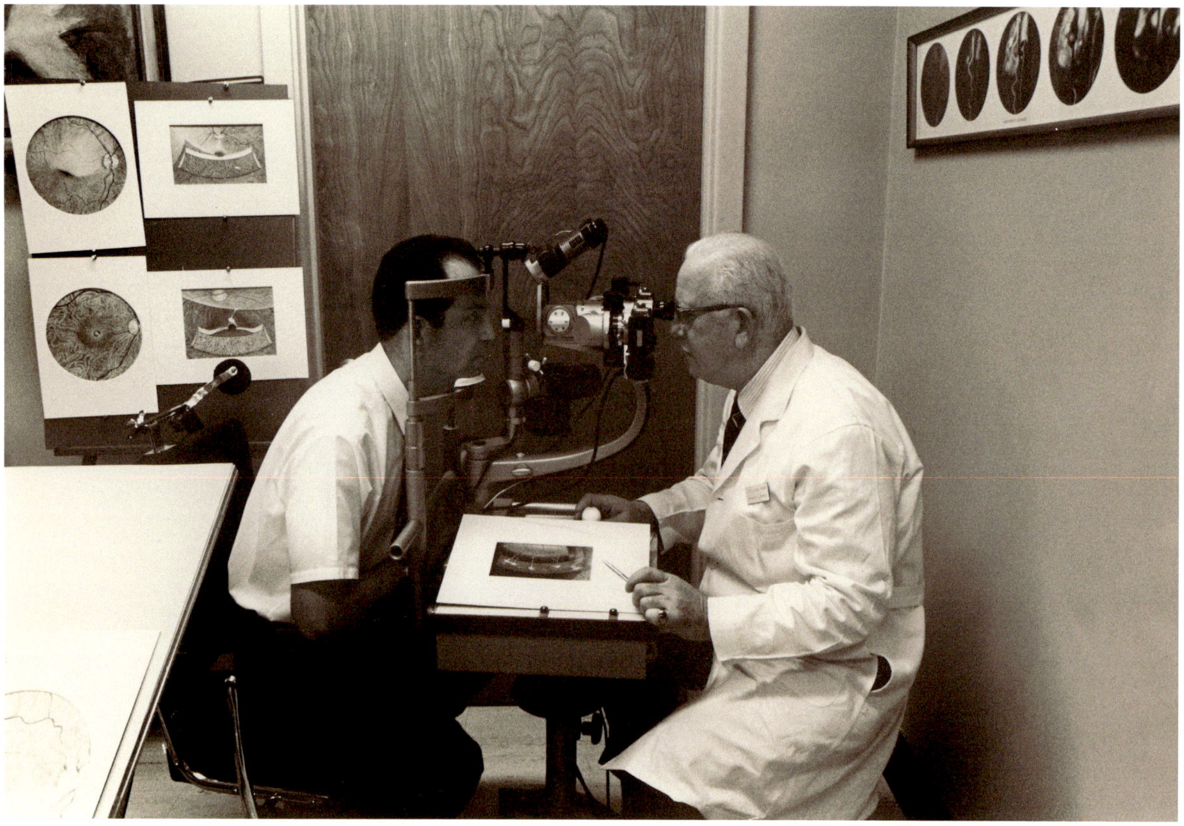

Fig. 3.

by the referring physician, on-site direct examination of the patient by use of the slit-lamp biomicroscope, the use of which he had apparently mastered while working with Berliner (Fig. 3), and consultation at the beginning, during and near completion to insure that his observations seemed correct (Fig. 4). From my observations and study of the paintings, Myers incorporated his own perception of the ocular findings, often enhancing and at times exaggerating features that emphasized the unique qualities, quantities, depth and location of the lesions. This use of "artistic license" is what captures the unique beauty of these magnificent illustrations, and hence the title of this publication—"An Artist's Perspective on the Eye." Examination of this art indicates that Myers used mixed media, including pencil sketches, oils and spray-airbrushing. The paintings are in either a round shape or a vertically rectangular format. Most of the round format measure 2 to 7 inches in diameter and the majority of the rectangular paintings are 3 x 6 inches, with many in a 4 x 6 to 7 inch format.

As far as I can determine, only one set of paintings were ever published in color, Plates 59, 60, and 61 were published by Gass and Norton in 1966.[1] Other publications which are in black and white include: Plates 15 and 16 by Luxenberg in 1967;[2] Plates 51, 52, 54a & b, 56 and 57 by Kasner et al. in 1968;[3] Plate 39 by Sever et al. in 1968;[4] Plates 60, 62b, 63b and 66 by Gass in 1970;[5] and Plate 88 by Curtin et al. in 1967.[6]

Fourteen of the paintings from seven patient diagnoses were obtained as a gift from Mr. Myers by James C. Major, MD, a former resident at the BPEI. After his death, his widow and son held these framed paintings. In 2008, his son James C. Major, Jr., Chief Resident at BPEI, brought the paintings to the Institute where they were removed from the frames, digitalized, reframed and returned to the Major family (Plates 12 to 16, 19 to 22, 25 to 28 and 31). The three paintings that were published in color (Plates 59, 60 and 61), are framed and in the possession of the Gass family, and were kindly loaned to us to be digitalized and reframed.

The descriptions of all the paintings have been made intentionally brief, to let the art "speak for itself."

Richard K. Forster, MD is Professor of Ophthalmology, Bascom Palmer Eye Institute
University of Miami Miller School of Medicine
The Richard K. Forster Chair in Corneal and External Diseases

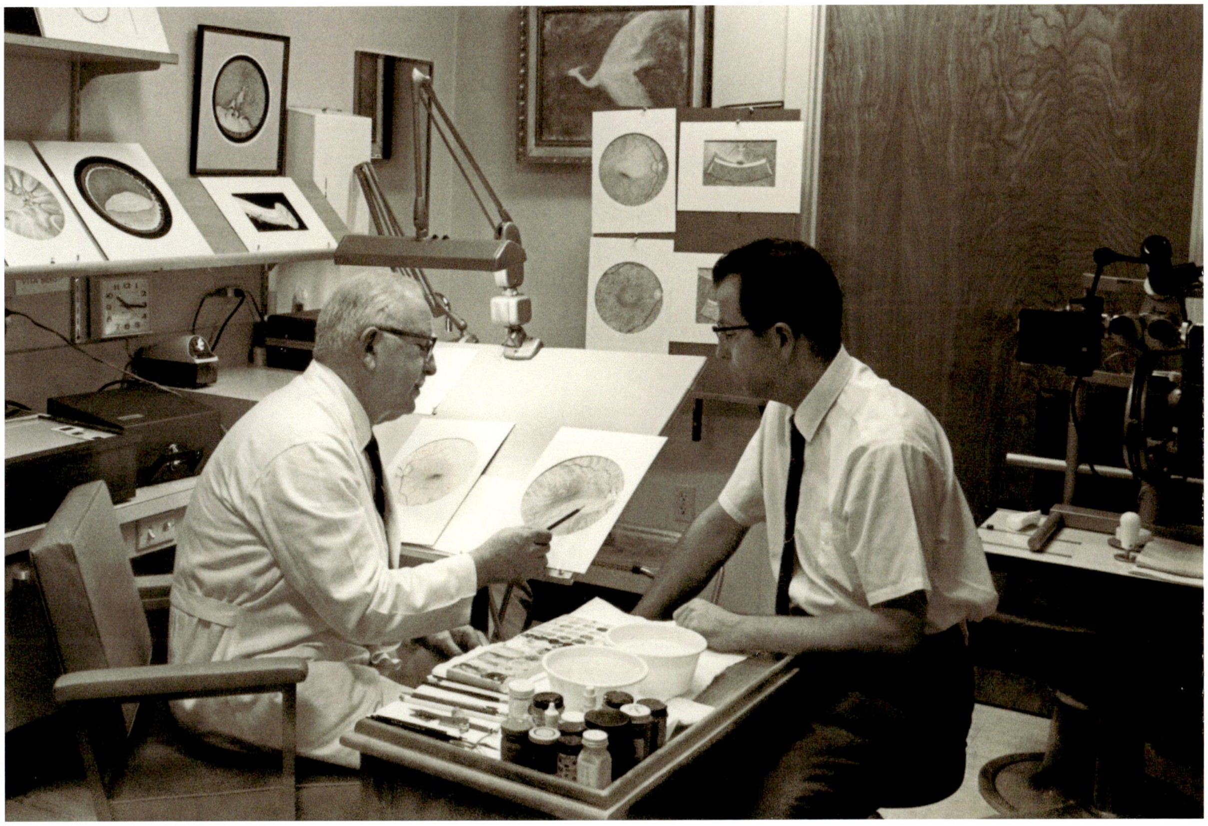

Fig. 4.

REFERENCES

1. Gass JDM, Norton EWD. Cystoid macular edema and papilledema following cataract extraction. Arch Ophthalmol 1966; 76:646-661.
2. Luxenberg M. Hereditary crystalline dystrophy of the cornea. Am J Ophthalmol 1967; 63:507-511.
3. Kasner D, Miller GR, Taylor WH, Sever RJ, Norton EWD. Surgical treatment of amyloidosis of the vitreous. Trans Am Acad Ophthalmol Otolaryngol 1968; 72:410-418.
4. Sever RJ, Frost P, Weinstein G. Eye changes in ichthyosis. JAMA 1968; 206:2283-2286.
5. Gass JDM. Stereoscopic Atlas of Macular Disease; a Funduscopic and Angiographic Presentation, 1st ed. St. Louis, CV Mosby, 1970.
6. Curtin VT, Norton EWD, Gass JDM. Photocoagulation: Its use in the prevention of reoperation after scleral buckling operations. Trans Am Acad Ophthalmol Otolaryngol 1967; 71:432-441.

Fig. 1:
Lattice Corneal Dystrophy
(see also plate 24)

Fig. 2a:
Clinical photograph of eye with Hereditary Crystalline Stromal Dystrophy of Schnyder

Fig. 2b:
Hereditary Crystalline Stromal Dystrophy of Schnyder
(see also plate 15)

Fig. 3:
Mr. Myers using the three-dimensional slit of the biomicroscope to observe the details of corneal pathology.

Fig. 4:
J. McGuinness Myers (left) in his studio on the fourth floor of the Bascom Palmer Eye Institute, conferring with Robert Machemer, MD.

FOREWORD

HELEN L. KOHEN, MIAMI, 2012

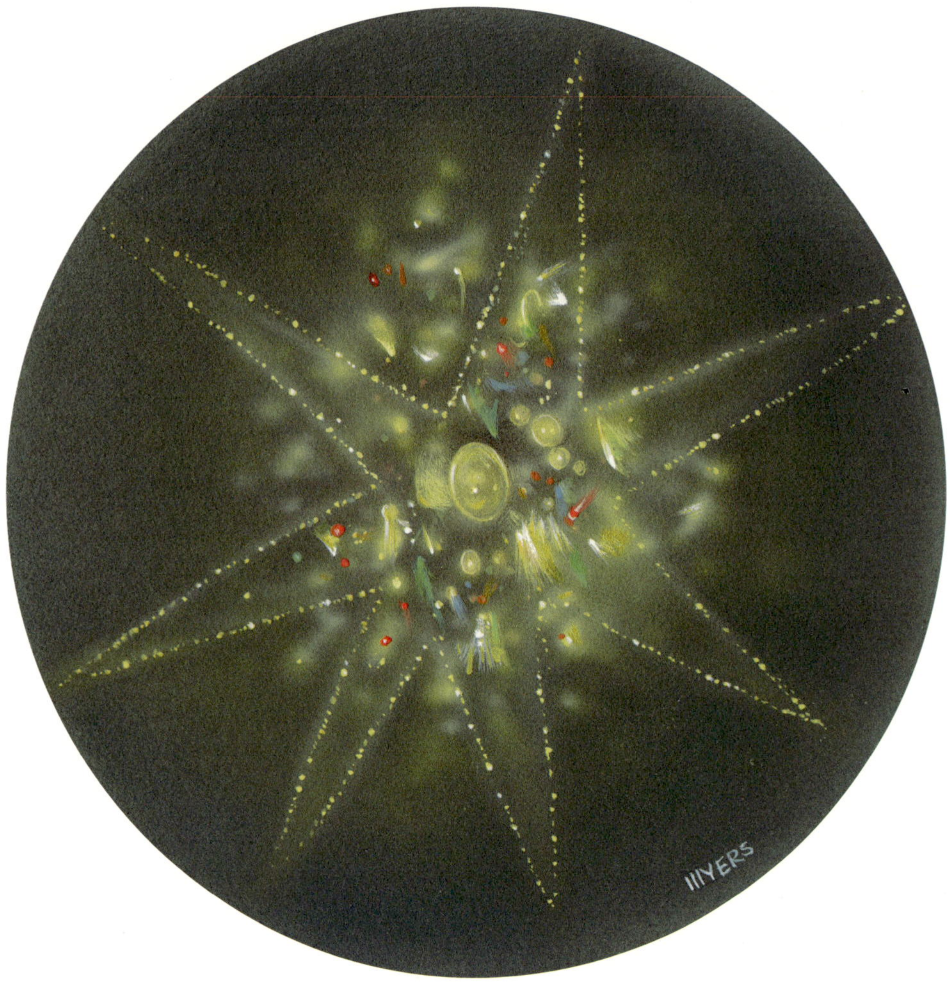

I'd venture that not too many art historians have the opportunity, much less the honor, of writing a foreword to a medical book. I am myself humbled by the concept, and also thrilled to play a small part in introducing the artwork of Jack McGuinness Myers to a community potentially greater than that of physicians and surgeons.

Indeed, though Myers was a medical illustrator by profession, the paintings and drawings he created on site at Bascom Palmer Eye Institute illuminating diseases of the eye would intrigue anyone attracted to fine art. That's precisely how Myers' pictures struck me when I first encountered them more than a year ago. It only seemed that I was in the wrong place for an art historian; it turned out that I was there for the right reason.

Invited by Dr. Richard Forster to "look over" a group of mounted mixed-media works on paper that illustrated medical conditions of the living eye, I was transported to other pictures in other places. I thought myself back in graduate school contemplating the origins of abstract art. There is one theory citing the source of the art style that goes like this: non-objective art (non-figurative, non-representational notions) were born of a long and fairly ancient tradition of limning the unknowable, making what cannot be seen visible to all as artworks. This group includes iterations on the occult, most especially visual expressions of the mysteries of the spiritual realm. Understand that all these images were created not from observed reality but in concert with the mind's eye. The attempts to illustrate Eastern philosophies formed a particular body of this sort of work. As those pictorial efforts were made manifest in thousands of examples, it was clear that pure and vivid color was a primary factor of expression, as was amorphous form. And this above all—that the outward shape these visions took was overwhelmingly circular—ocular.

There, in the handsome library of the Bascom Palmer Eye Institute, I was viewing similar images, albeit they were actually exactingly scientific, carefully articulated medical illustrations of the human eye. As familiar as I thought I was with anatomical material, this was a revelation. I was immediately drawn into Dr. Forster's own enthusiasm for Myers' exquisite renderings and became a champion of the doctor's desire to see them properly published. It would be a volume of special interest to eye doctors but—and this is my bias—the illustrations might delight every casual visitor to its pages.

Myers worked at Bascom Palmer from 1966 to 1968, the last two years of his life, creating just over one hundred works. Well celebrated as a medical illustrator of the eye—his work was featured in two major tomes on the subject in the 1940s—the artist painted just those abnormalities that were found in patients during his tenure at the Institute. Thus this book is no comprehensive compendium of the possible diseases of the eye, but merely a survey of those that Myers encountered during a specific period of time. The artist was aided in his observations by various instruments, microscopes, photographs, special lighting, and of course the cooperation of the patients and faculty of Bascom Palmer.

Still, the variety of his subject matter coupled with his facility with paints, pencil, air-brush and ink is stunning to see. The finished works are immaculate, worthy of the technical skills of a miniaturist. The layman, ignorant of the medical details each picture is provided with, might spin any number of narratives from what is seen on the pages of "An Artist's Perspective on the Eye." There are what appear to be Op Art designs, diminishing vistas and swelling curves, images of swimming fish and even the suggestion of dancing flowers. The colors range from muted to dazzling, every picture a study of tone and color value. One illustration (opposite page and Plate 48), identified as the 'Christmas tree cataract,' looks like a holiday ornament, a free-hand star with pinpoint lights ablaze. A few of the paintings appear to represent perfect circles of celestial brightness, and one, illuminating the case of a melanoma of the retina, might be taken for a Japanese landscape (Plate 83).

Which is not to diminish the worth of "An Artist's Perspective on the Eye" as a valuable medical book, nor to turn the tables on the expectations of art lovers. My single role in this enterprise is to aid in the celebration of Myers as a significant artist, to champion his work sufficiently to potentiate its preservation, and to help in handing it off to all those who would find it meaningful. And, in fact, the works speak for themselves. Dr. Forster and Dr. Edward Norton before him knew it all well before I came on the scene: Myers' paintings have been cataloged and cherished by Bascom Palmer Eye Institute for more than forty-four years. This volume only insures that Myers' treasured illustrations (along with the accompanying text) will find a degree of permanency, and that many more than those doctors privy to its former archival existence will have the opportunity to learn from it and enjoy its pleasures.

PLATES 1 – 4

Epidemic Keratoconjunctivitis (EKC): Progression of Corneal Stages

These paintings beautifully illustrate the classic sequence of corneal changes that are virtually diagnostic of this highly contagious viral disease. Mr. Myers made these paintings at the request of D.B. Jones, MD, at the time a resident at the Bascom Palmer Eye Institute and currently the Chairman of the Cullen Eye Institute in Houston, Texas, who provided sketches to Mr. Myers. They are generic in the sense that they are not taken from examination of a specific patient over time, but rather to demonstrate the sequence and progression of the corneal changes in the viral syndrome of EKC.

PLATE 1

Punctate Epithelial Erosions

A myriad of diffuse fine clear punctate epithelial erosions appear about five to seven days after the onset of symptoms. Also, about four to five days after the first corneal manifestation, the fellow eye develops similar lesions, but usually to a lesser degree.

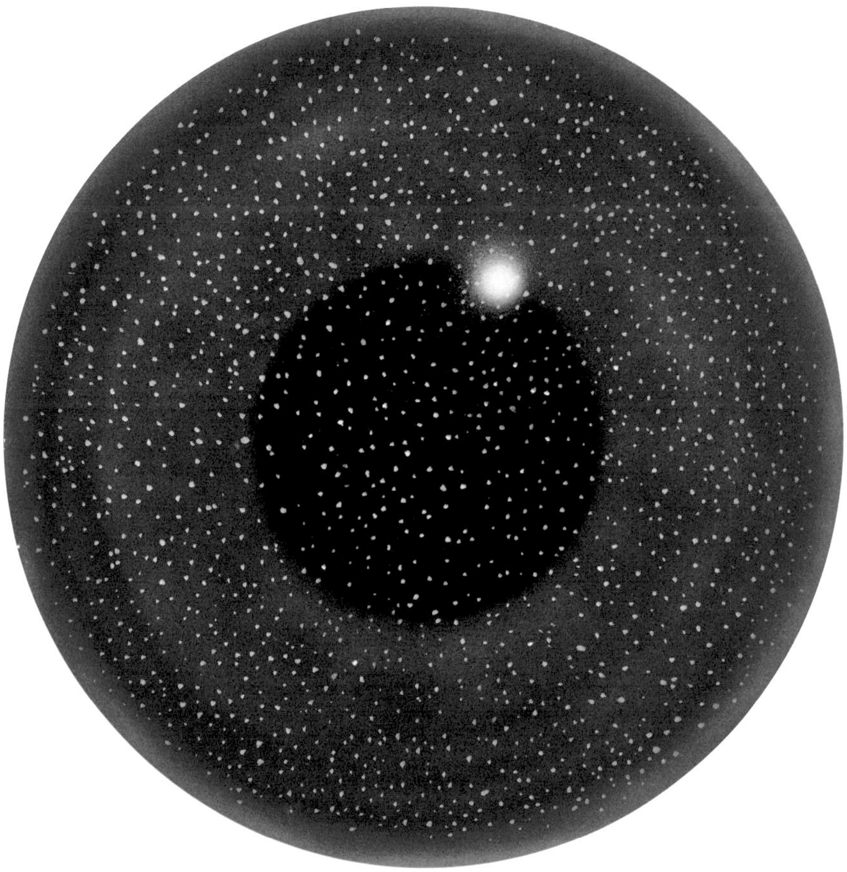

1a

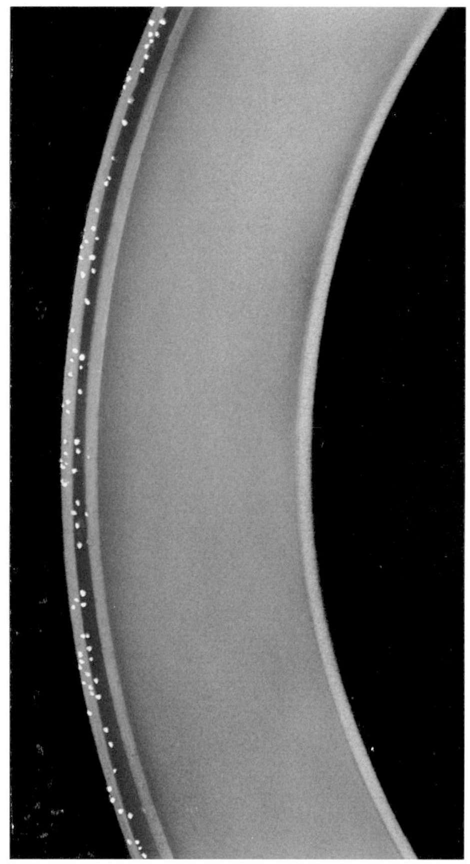

1b

PLATE 2

Punctate Epithelial Keratitis

After another four to five days, the fine erosions begin to dissipate and coalesce into slightly elevated clumps taking on a focal opacity which represents the transition to the second stage of the keratitis. The configuration and shape of these lesions is a punctate epithelial keratitis, which includes a mild corneal inflammatory response with the lesions larger than those in the initial stages.

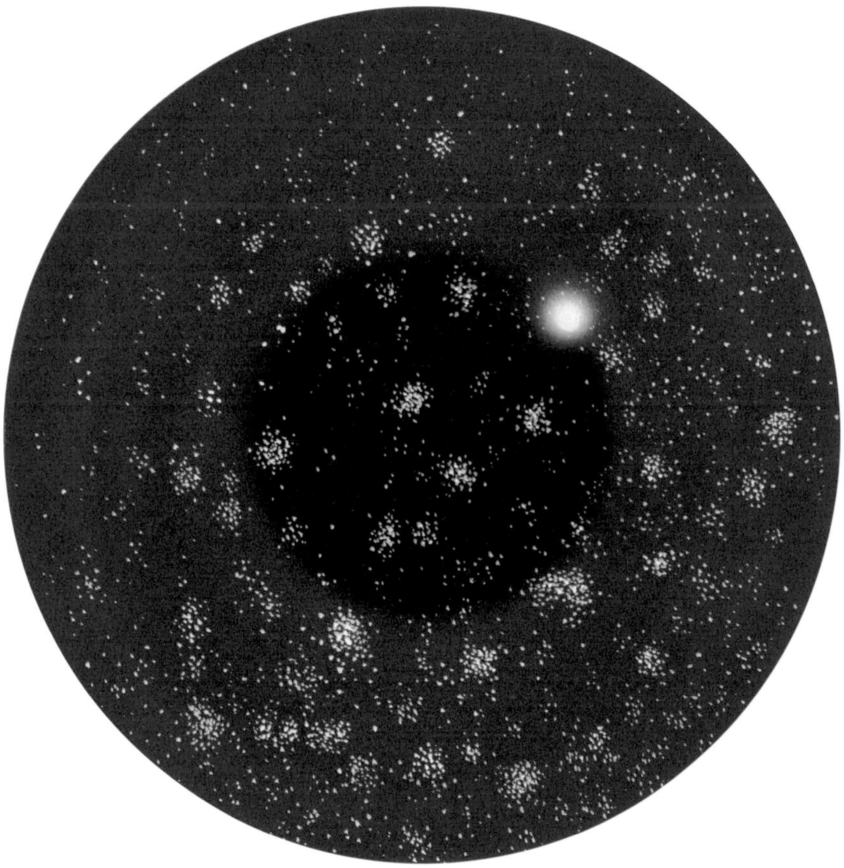

2a

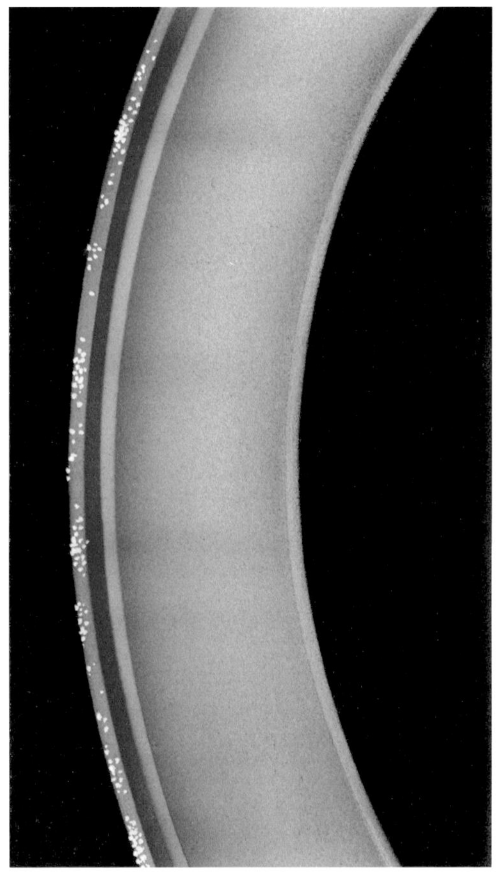

2b

PLATE 3

Transitional Stage of the Corneal Changes of Epidemic Keratoconjunctivitis

This transitional stage is characterized by discrete localized punctate epithelial lesions beginning to involve the deeper level of the basement membrane and initiates the development of the third stage of the keratitis: punctate subepithelial infiltrates.

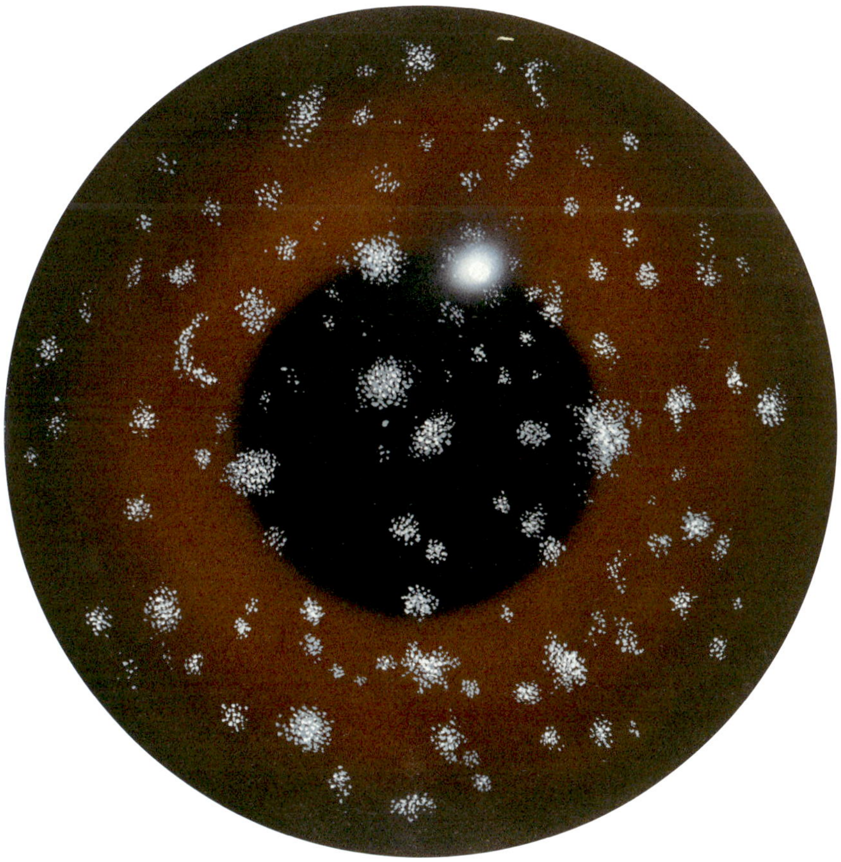

3a

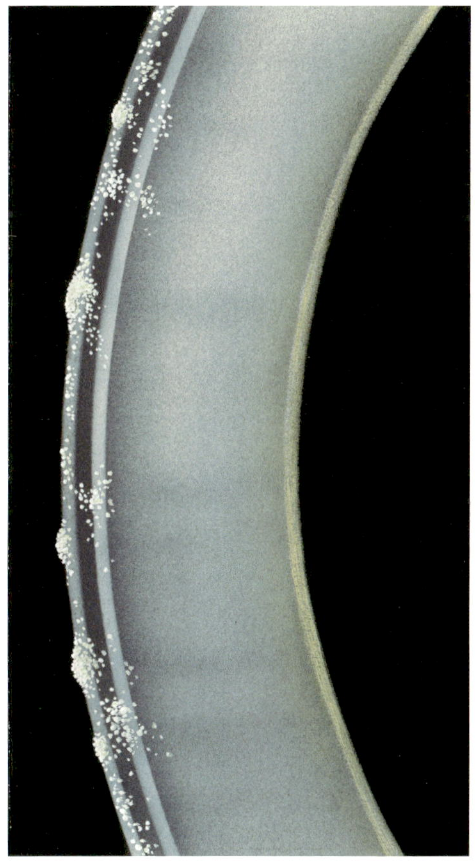

3b

PLATE 4

Punctate Subepithelial Infiltrates

By about two weeks after the initial corneal changes appear, the superficial punctate lesions disappear and the immune-related inflammation is transferred to the superficial level of Bowman layer beneath the epithelial basement membrane, forming discrete reticulated or net-like nummular opacities referred to as punctate subepithelial infiltrates. These opacities remain for weeks, months, and often up to two or more years, usually affecting vision if the lesions involve the visual axis.

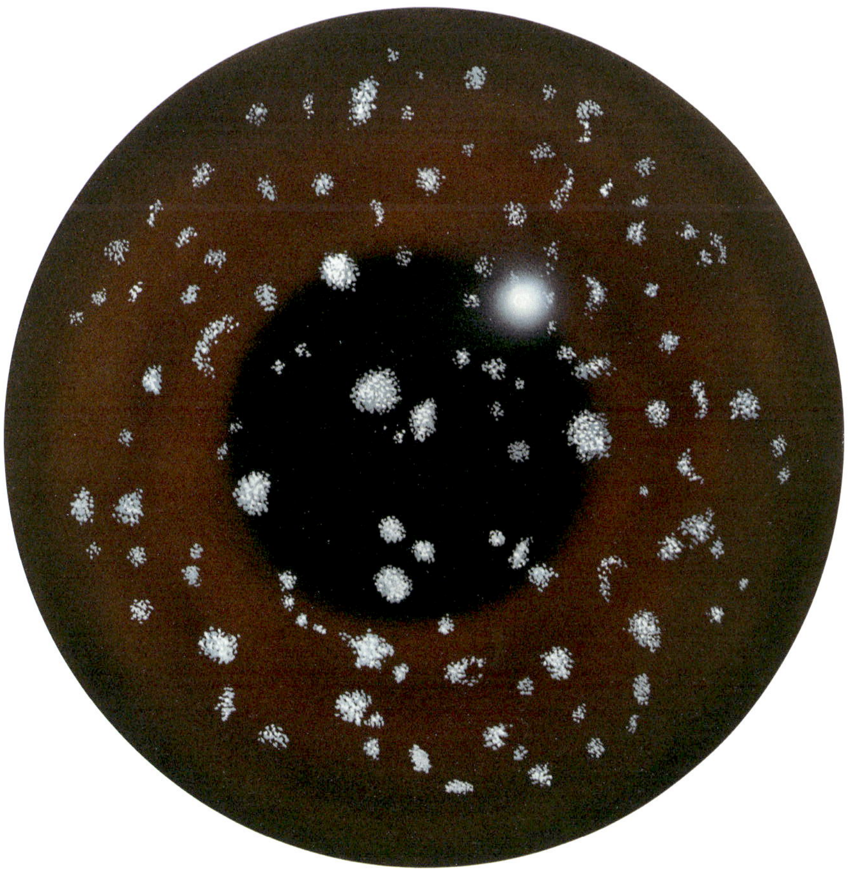

4a

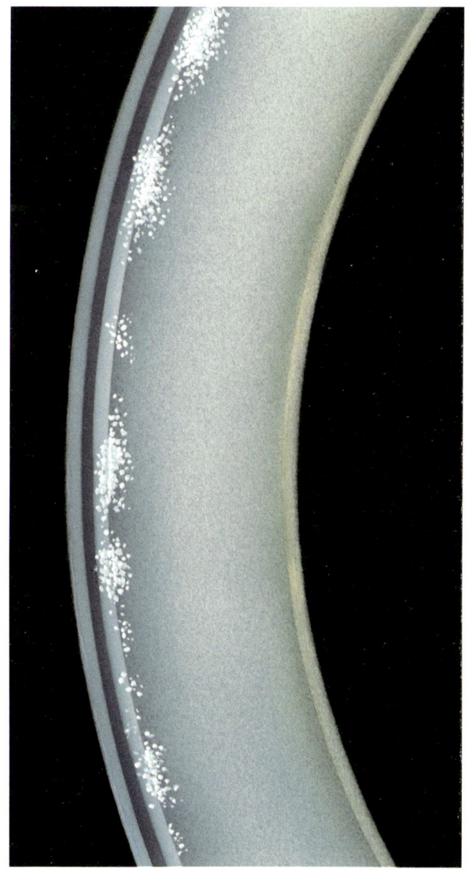

4b

PLATES 5 & 6

Epithelial Basement Membrane Dystrophy

These paintings illustrate either an inherited corneal dystrophy or more likely, a corneal degeneration due to repeated recurrent or chronic epithelial surface disease involving predominantly the basement membrane of the corneal epithelium. In the BPEI archives, this painting is labeled as a "Meesmann-type" or "Whorl Dystrophy," and probably represents a variant of Epithelial Basement Membrane Dystrophy.

PLATE 5

The laminar or reduplicated material seems localized to the subepithelial basement membrane and does not appear to involve the superficial Bowman zone beneath. There are several recognized variants of epithelial basement membrane dystrophy, mainly map-like changes, fingerprint-like lines or dots. In addition, the variant referred to as Stocker-Holt involves the anterior cornea diffusely, with opacities that appear in a whorl pattern; variants of Meesmann Corneal Dystrophy could result in this appearance over time.

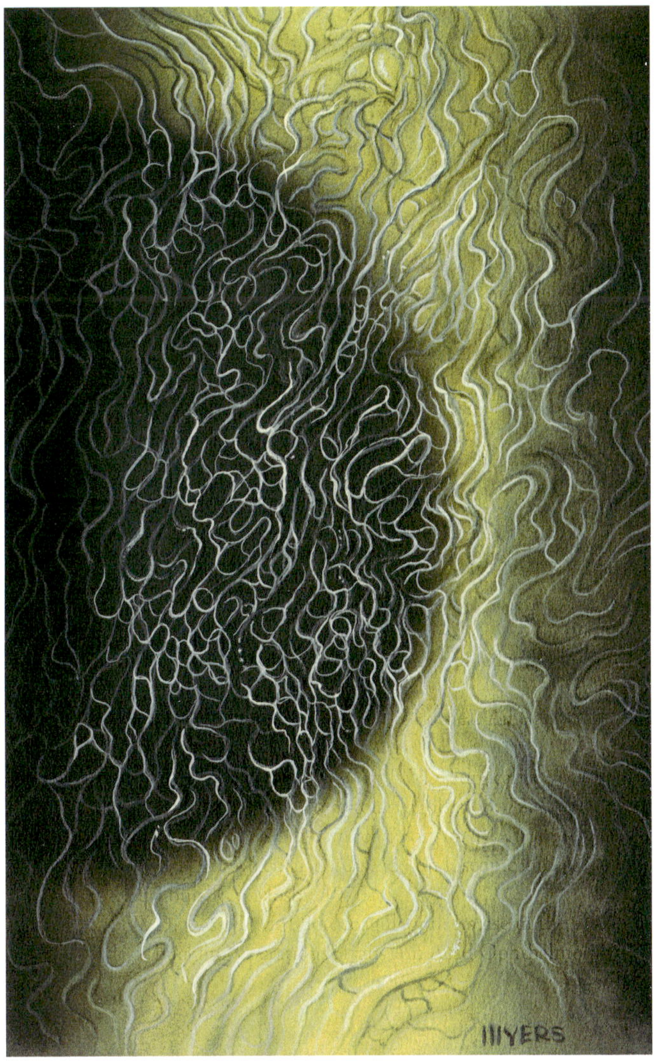

5a

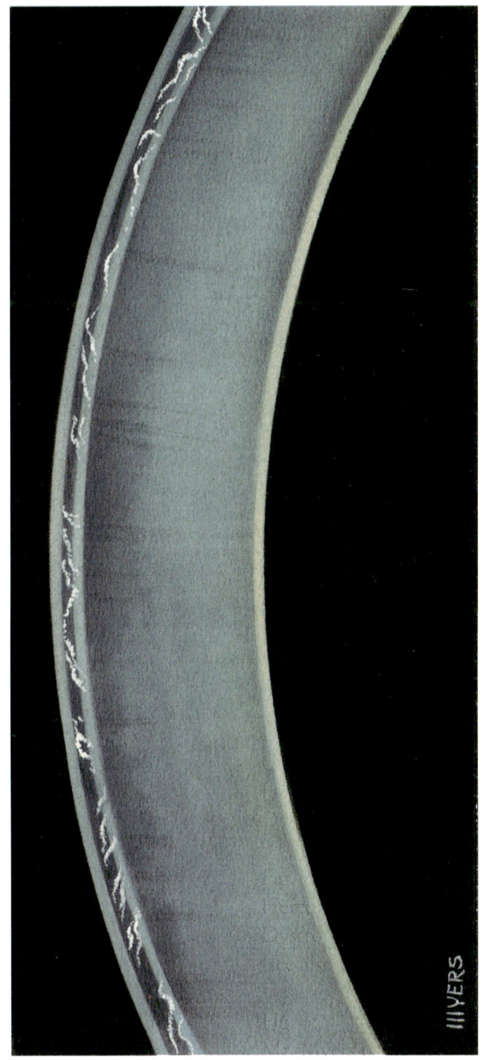

5b

PLATE 6

This painting is from the same patient as illustrated in Plate 5 a and b, but in this retroilluminated view with the background light reflecting off the retina, the changes appear more homogeneous and bleb-like. Such a pattern is recognized as a variant of Epithelial Basement Membrane Dystrophy. As with most corneal degenerations in contrast to corneal dystrophies which are inherited corneal diseases, the pattern of corneal changes are often more variable and open to interpretation. The term Cogan Microcystic Epithelial Dystrophy has also been used to describe variants of map-dot-fingerprint and Meesmann Corneal Dystrophy. Following a lecture at the Bascom Palmer Eye Institute by Dr. David Cogan in the early 1980s, I asked him what condition he described in Cogan's Microcystic Dystrophy and he interrupted to say that others had named it after him. I then qualified the question by asking whether he was describing the corneal changes of Meesmann dystrophy or the dot-form of Epithelial Basement Membrane Dystrophy, to which he replied, "I don't know which I was describing."

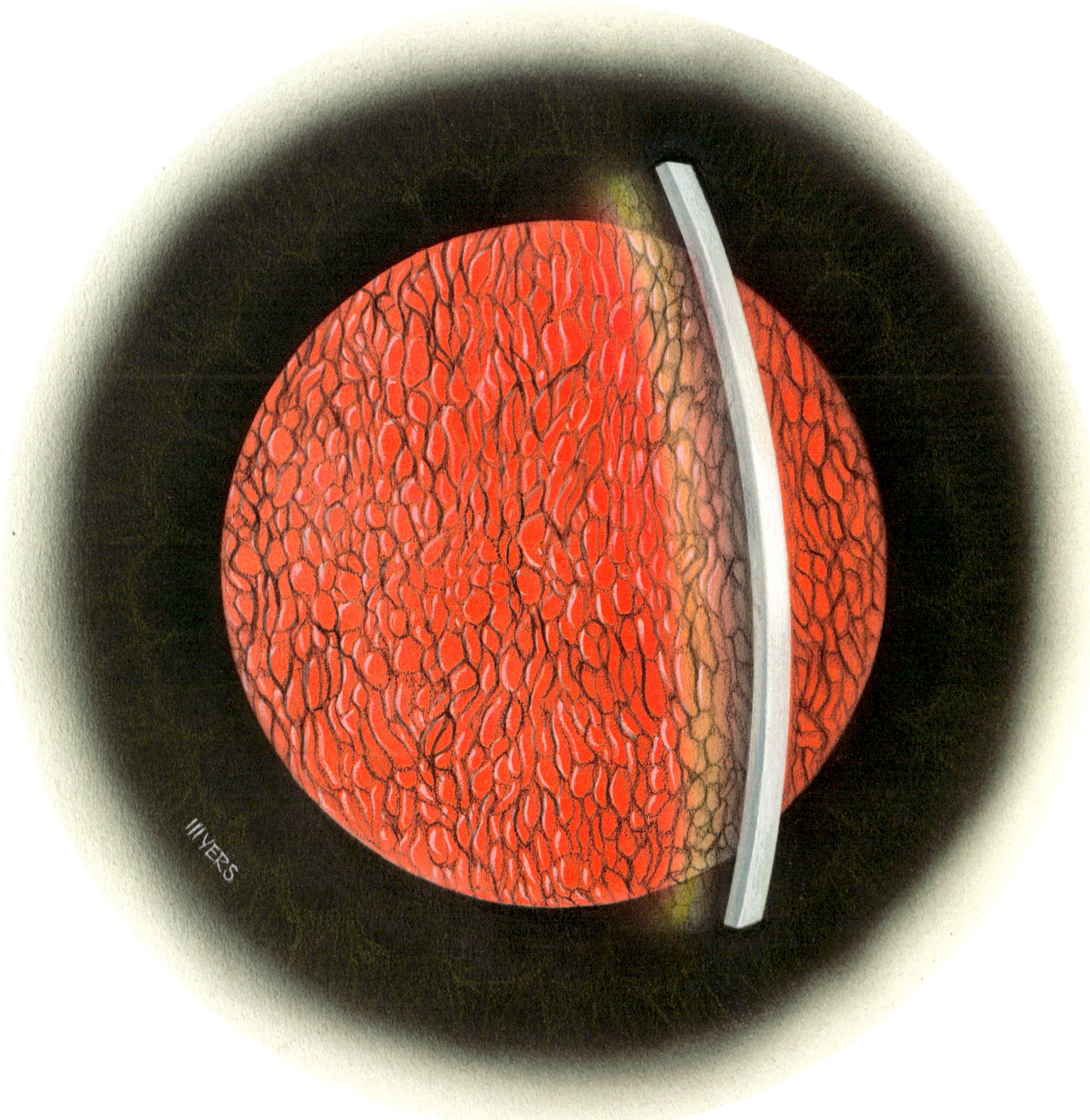
MYERS

PLATE 7

Bleb-Pattern Variant of Epithelial Basement Membrane Dystrophy

The title of these two paintings in the Bascom Palmer Eye Institute archives is Cogan's Microcystic Dystrophy. Examination of the paintings illustrates bleb-like subepithelial changes at the level of the basement membrane of the epithelium (7a). The sclerotic scatter view, with some retroillumination as demonstrated in 7b, shows diffuse cobblestone-like or a crocodile shagreen pattern typical of the bleb dystrophy variant of Epithelial Basement Membrane Dystrophy. In my experience, the blebs appear contiguous to each other centrally and somewhat more sparse in the mid-periphery, as if some of the "cobblestones" were missing or removed.

It is of note, that on the back of the paper mounted on board painting (7b), Mr. Myers indicated that "the lesions appear larger on retroillumination," and he apparently painted them thusly.

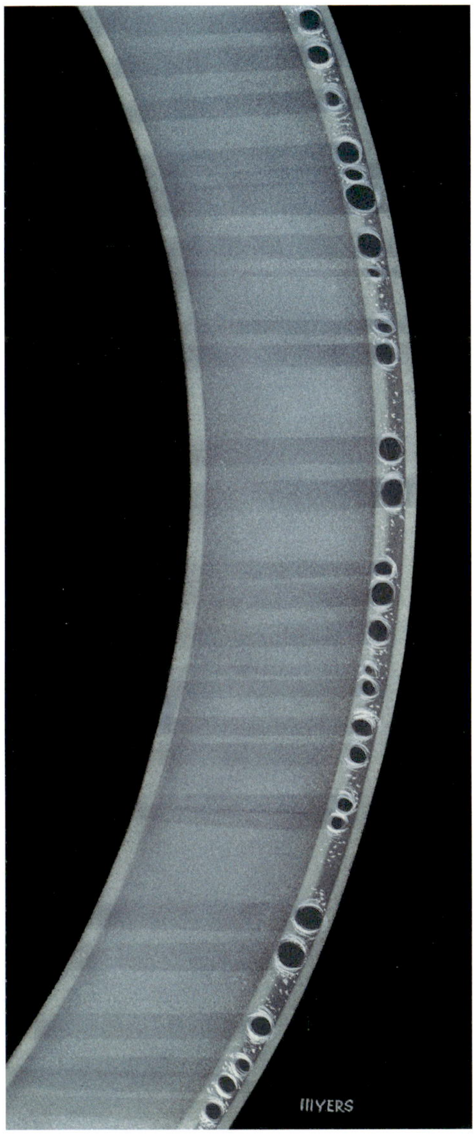

7a

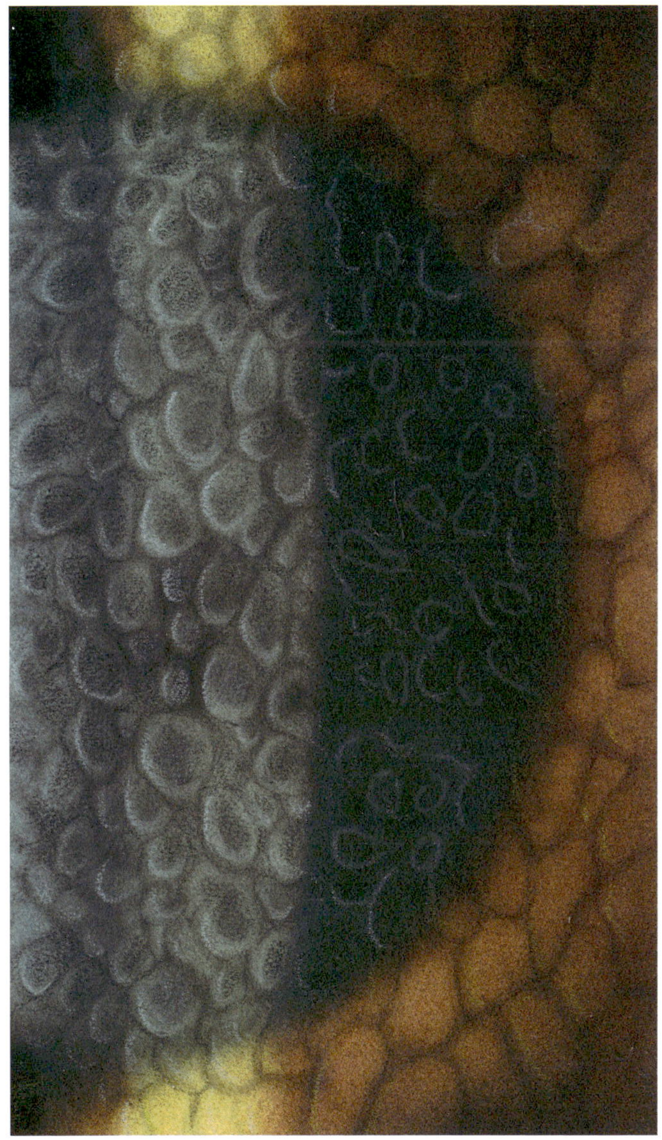

7b

PLATES 8 & 9

Calcific Keratopathy

This condition represents a corneal degeneration with deposition of calcium in the superficial cornea, usually localized to the level of the basement membrane of the epithelium and sometimes deeper at the superficial layer of Bowman zone.

PLATE 8

Although in this painting the changes diffusely involve the whole cornea, more often the entity is referred to as calcific band-shaped keratopathy, with the calcium deposited in a "band" horizontally across the cornea in the palpebral fissure area between the partially closed lids. Characteristically, the keratopathy appears as a dusky-grey deposition with "Swiss cheese"-like clear areas, thought to be the site of superficial corneal nerves. In systemic hypercalcemia, the deposition can be diffuse over most of the corneal surface, as in this painting. The band-shaped pattern is more often associated with chronic intraocular inflammation, although it is often of unknown etiology.

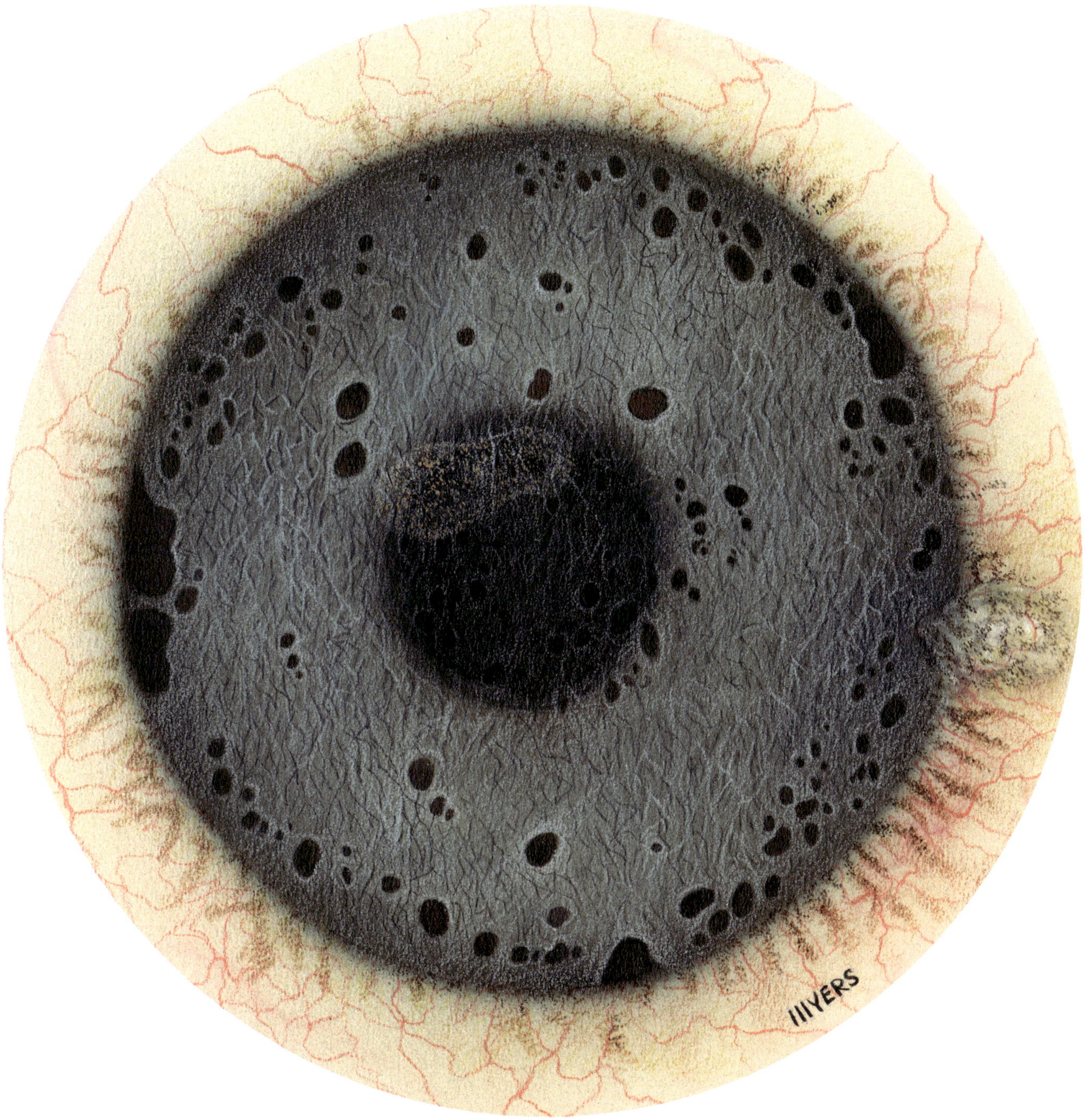
MYERS

PLATE 9

This 3-dimensional slit-beam view demonstrates the location of the calcium deposition at the level of the basement membrane and superficial Bowman zone. The Swiss-cheese configuration is highlighted. Most of the calcium can be removed, especially in the central and mid-periphery of the cornea, and if the deposition is superficial, by a mechanical/chemical process called chelation.

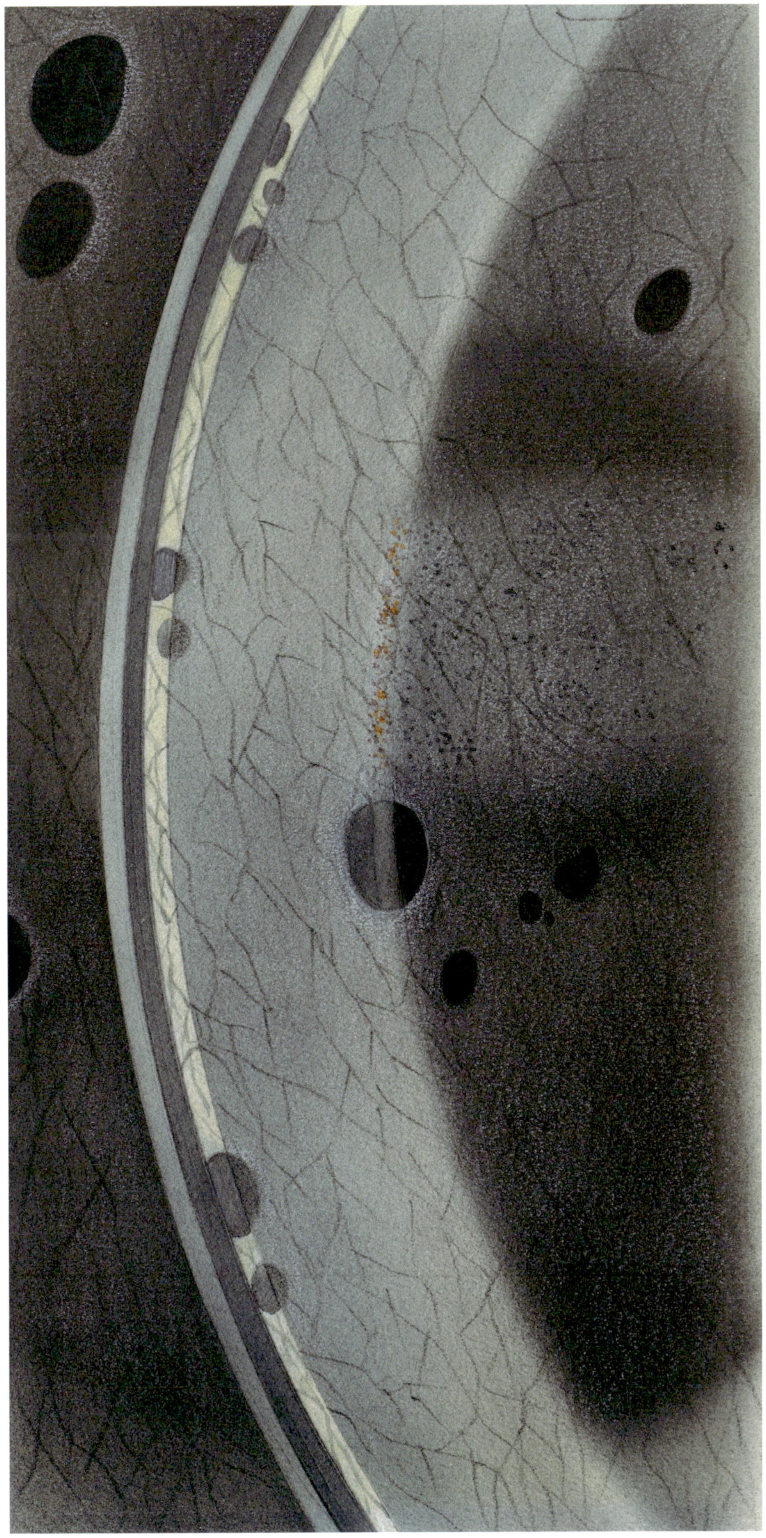

PLATES 10 & 11

Reis-Bücklers Corneal Dystrophy

PLATE 10

An autosomal dominantly inherited dystrophy involving the superficial stroma of the cornea at the level of Bowman layer. This dystrophy, with a genetic locus at 5q31, is also referred to as Corneal Dystrophy of Bowman layer type I (CDB-I).

It is characterized by confluent, but often irregular, geographic-like opacities often in a molten-glass or whorl configuration. The location is at the level of the superficial corneal stroma in the area referred to as Bowman layer or zone. With time, the lesions increase in area, density and depth.

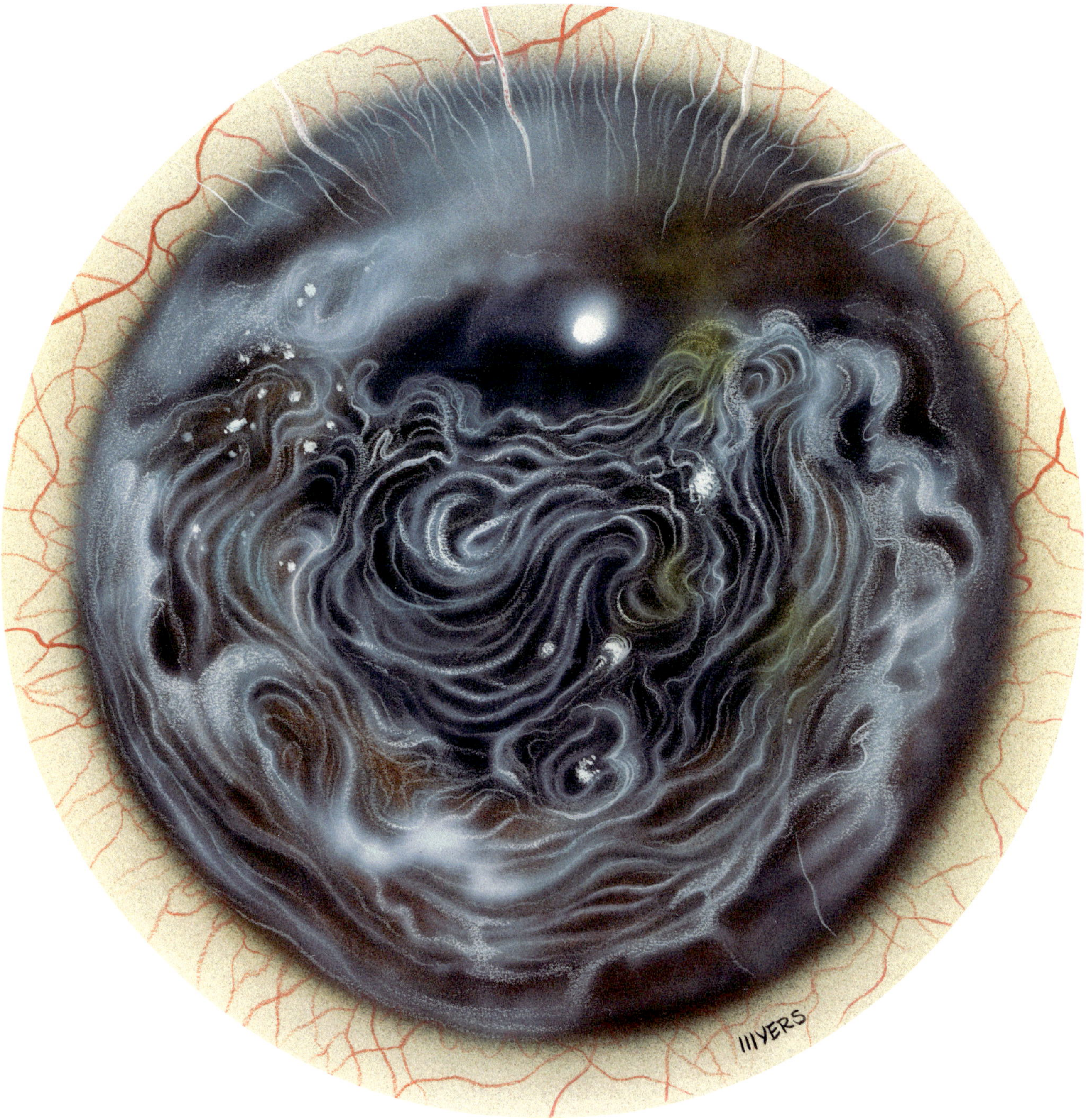
MYERS

PLATE 11

A slit-beam view with some retroillumination and a dilated pupil demonstrates the level of the opacity in the superficial stroma. As with most inherited corneal dystrophies, the lesions tend to be axial, thus leading to decreased vision earlier, but often increasing in area with time. Because of the superficial corneal irregularity and decreased vision, patients can often be helped visually by contact lens fitting, which may defer the need for surgery. Unfortunately, after surgery, there is a high likelihood of recurrence.

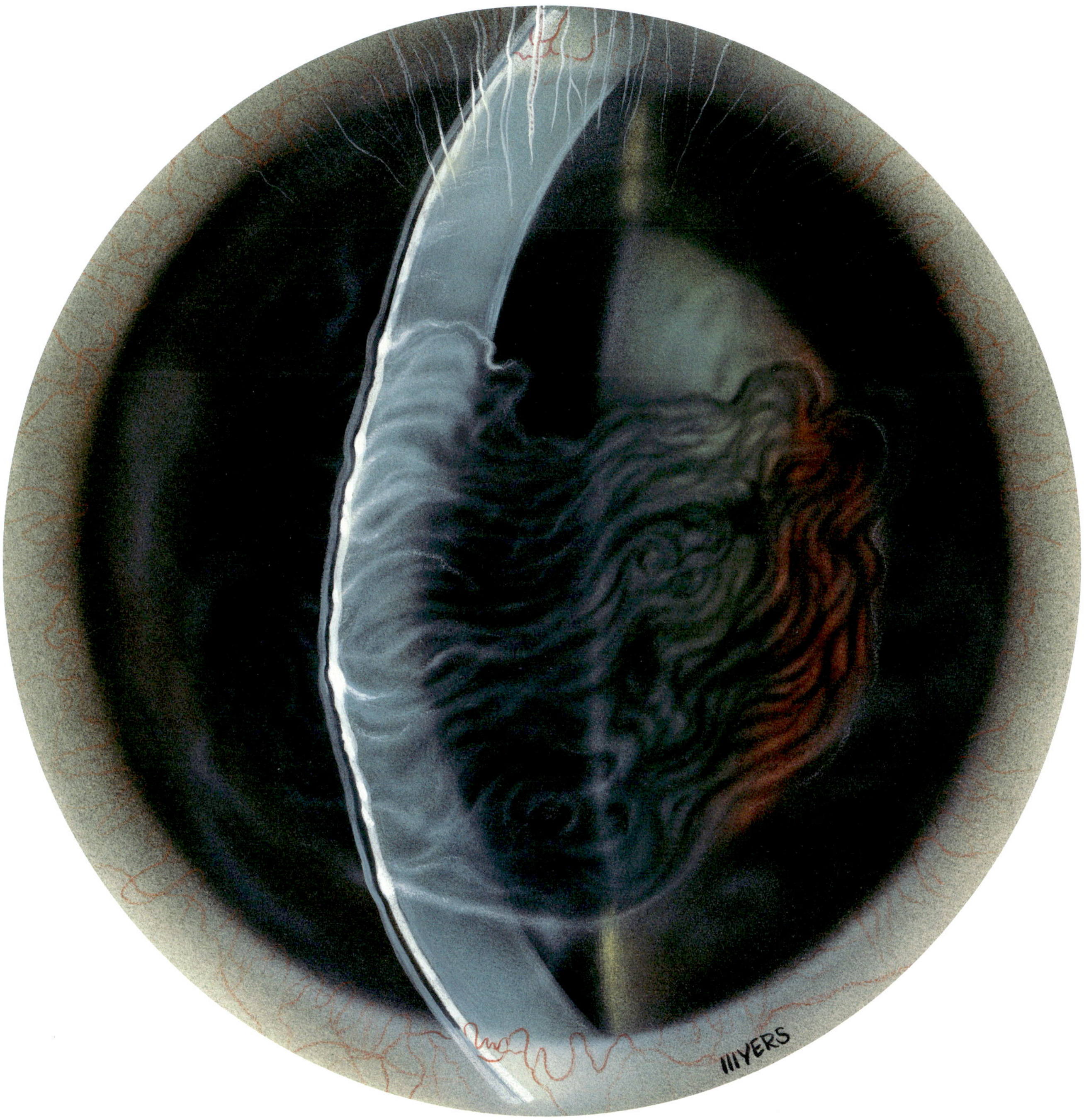
MYERS

PLATES 12 – 14

Thiel-Behnke Corneal Dystrophy

An autosomal dominantly inherited corneal dystrophy, genetically almost identical to Reis-Bücklers dystrophy (Plates 10 and 11), with the genetic locus at 5q31 and 10q24. Recently, it has been referred to as Corneal Dystrophy of Bowman layer type II (CDB-II). It is characterized by a subepithelial honeycomb pattern of opacities at the superficial stroma at the level of Bowman layer.

PLATE 12

Beautifully illustrated, with the opacities at the superficial layer of the stroma and the slit-lamp light reflecting off the iris and lens to demonstrate the honeycomb, anterior "crocodile-shagreen" pattern. In this case, the opacities had progressed to the corneal periphery. It is likely that this patient had recurrent corneal erosions resulting in the focal subepithelial scars.

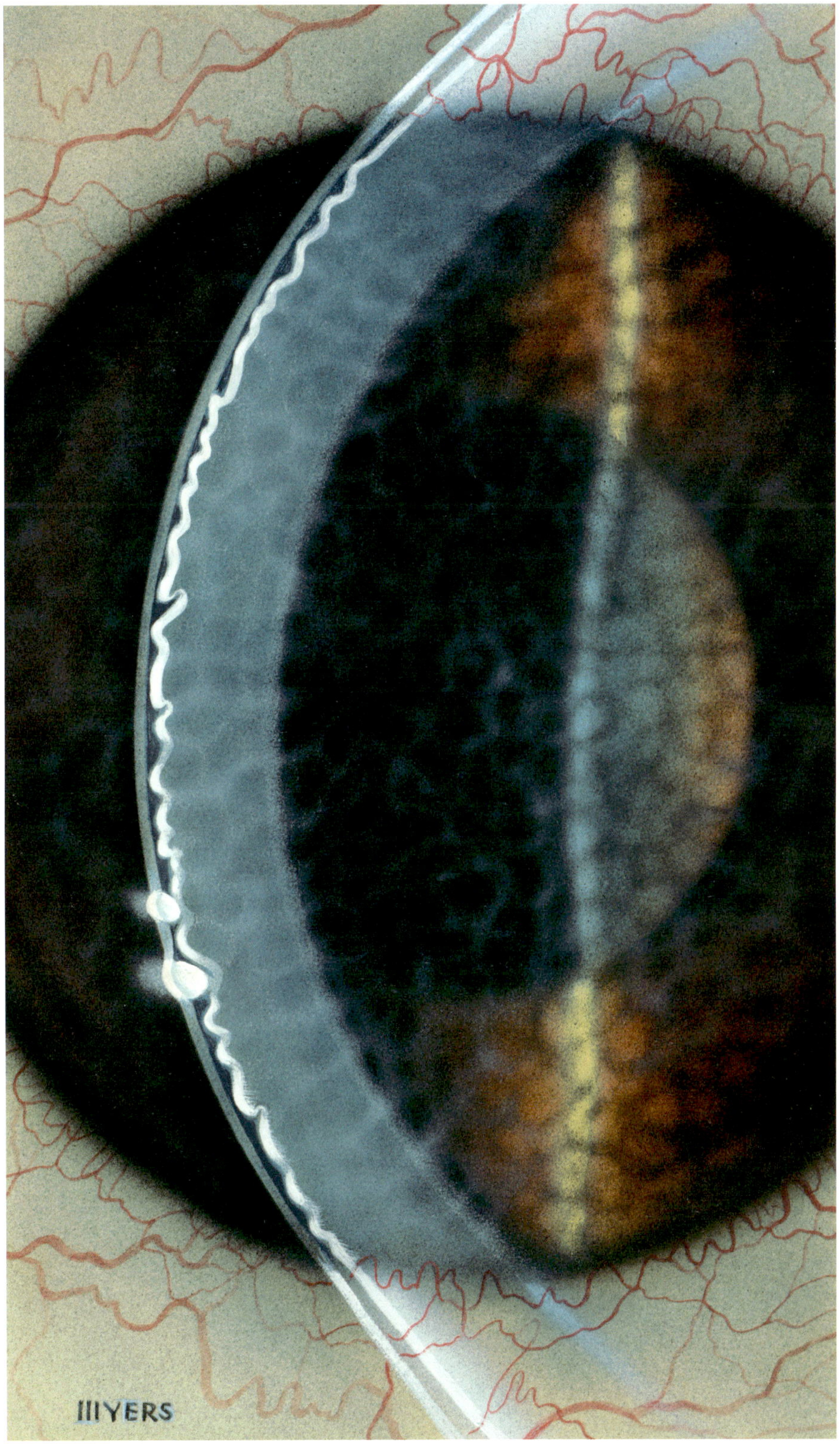
MYERS

PLATE 13

This painting illustrates the reticulated pattern under increased magnification with the technique of sclerotic-scatter, which aids in this partial retroillumination view.

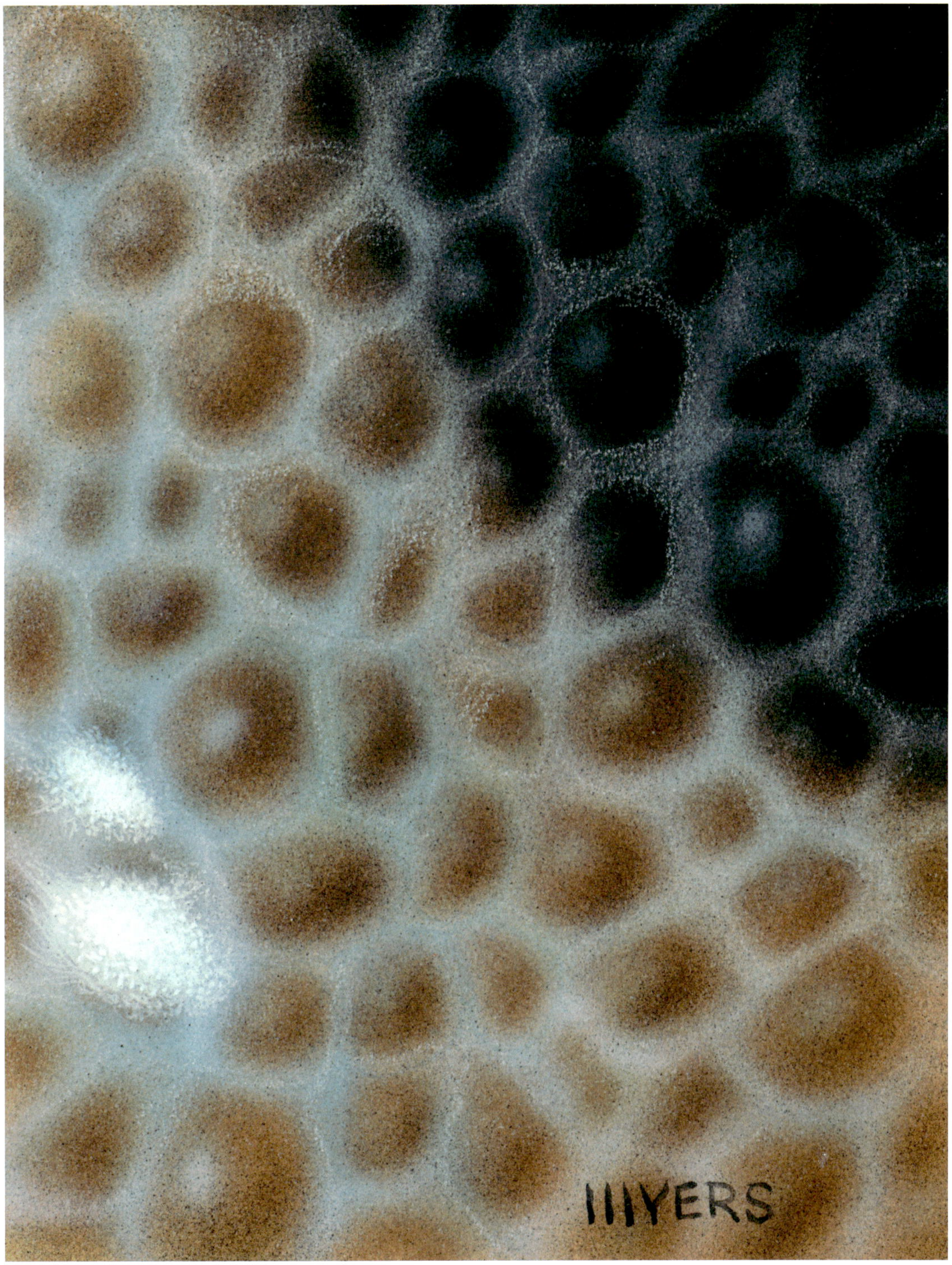
MYERS

PLATE 14

The honeycomb pattern is evident by retroillumination, with the two subepithelial opacities seen in silhouette.

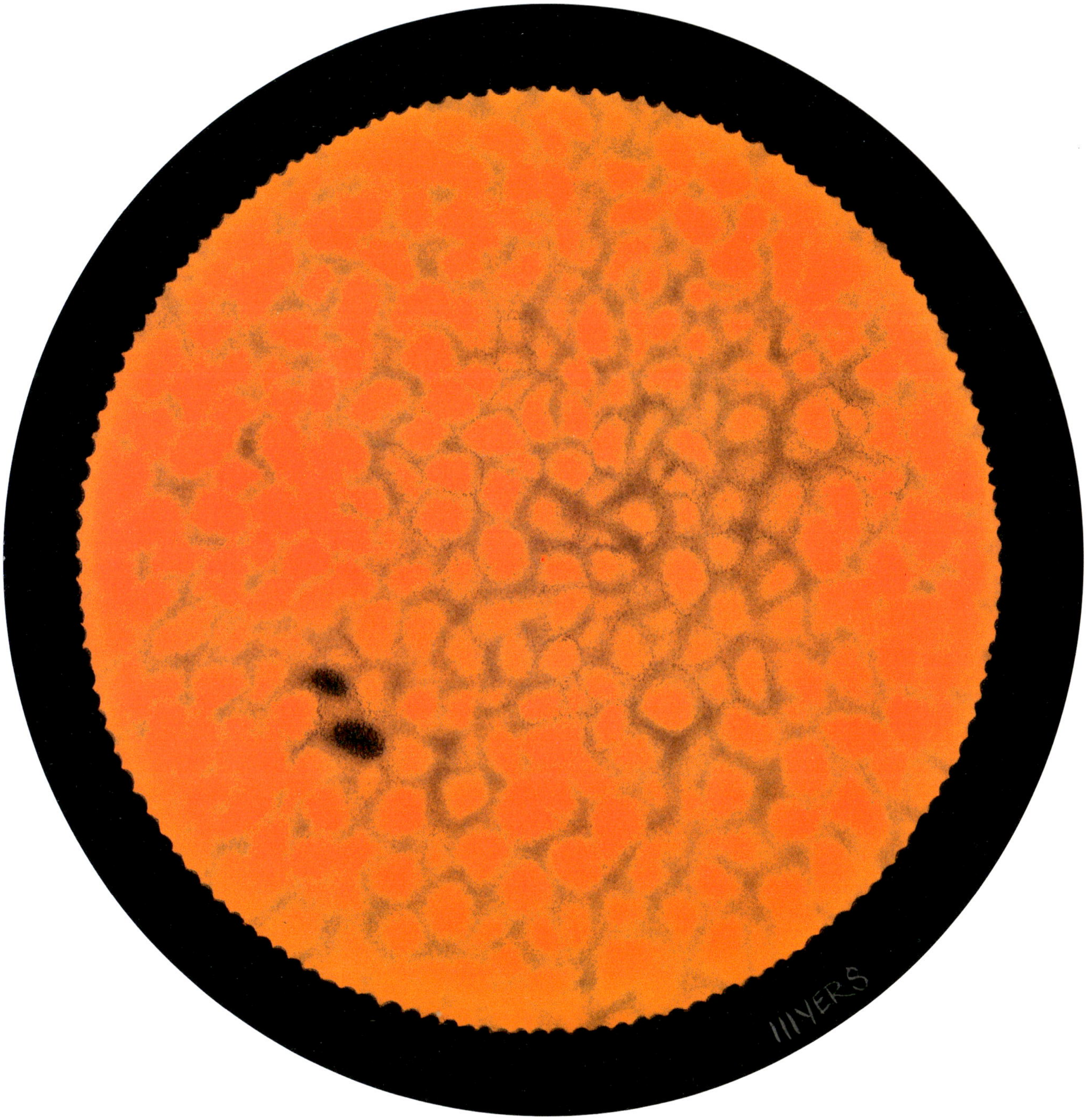

PLATES 15 & 16

Hereditary Crystalline Stromal Dystrophy of Schnyder

An autosomal dominant stromal dystrophy often with a delayed diagnosis until the corneal crystals become associated with a peripheral arcus and stromal haze, or if diagnosed earlier in life, with a family history of this diagnosis. This entity is characterized by abnormal intracellular and extracellular deposition of phospholipids and cholesterol.

These two plates were published in black and white in an article by Malcolm Luxenberg, MD in 1967, following his residency training at the Bascom Palmer Eye Institute. (Luxenberg M. Hereditary crystalline dystrophy of the cornea. Am J Ophthalmol 1967; 63:507-511)

PLATE 15

Central island of slightly polychromatic crystals in the subepithelium and anterior stroma, associated with a peripheral arcus lipoides.

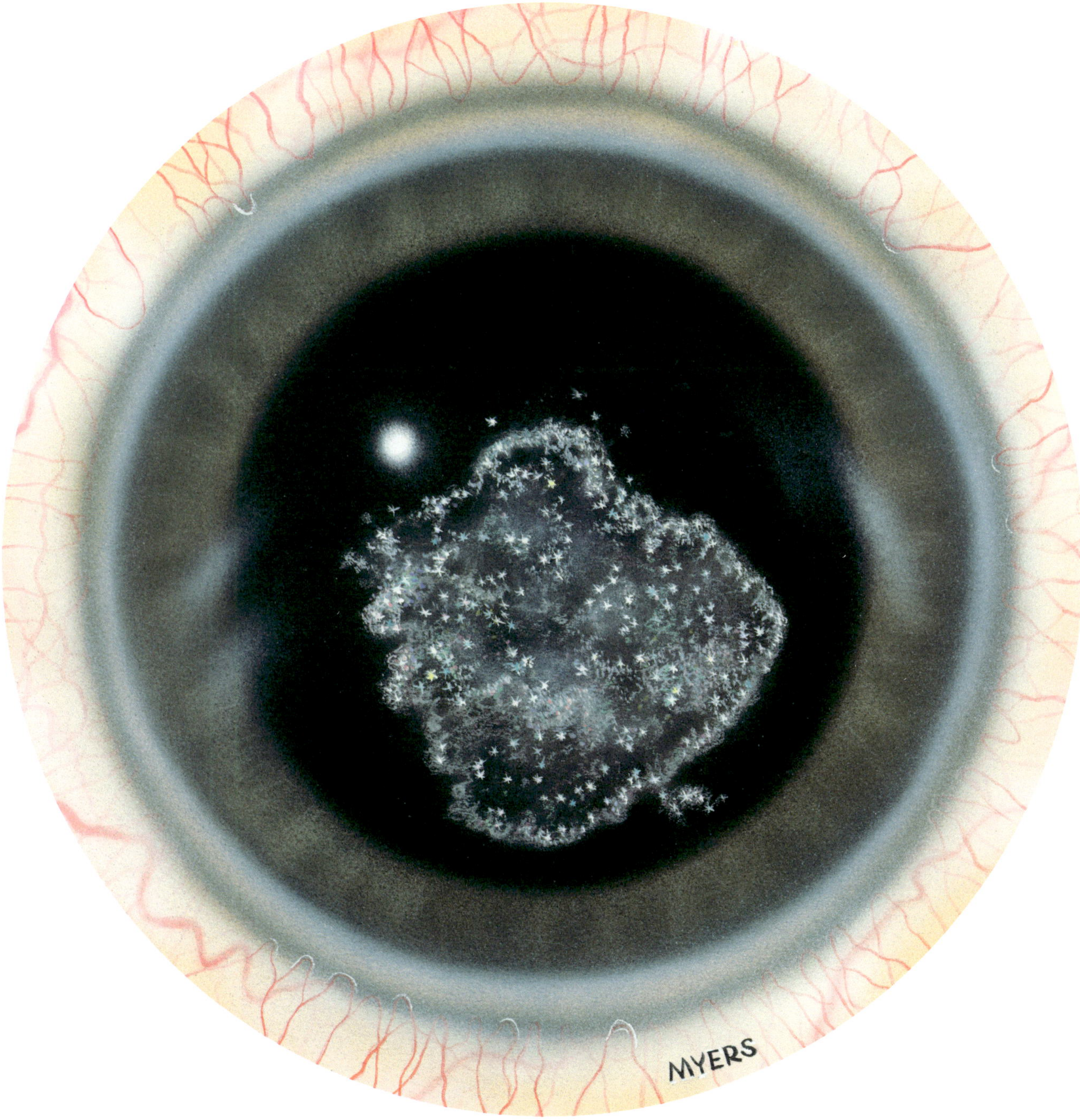
MYERS

PLATE 16

This slit-beam view demonstrates that the crystals are primarily located in the subepithelial Bowman layer and anterior stroma. The peripheral arcuate fatty opacity is typical and is characterized by deposition of lipids in the superficial and deep stroma, with a clear zone in the extreme periphery of the cornea.

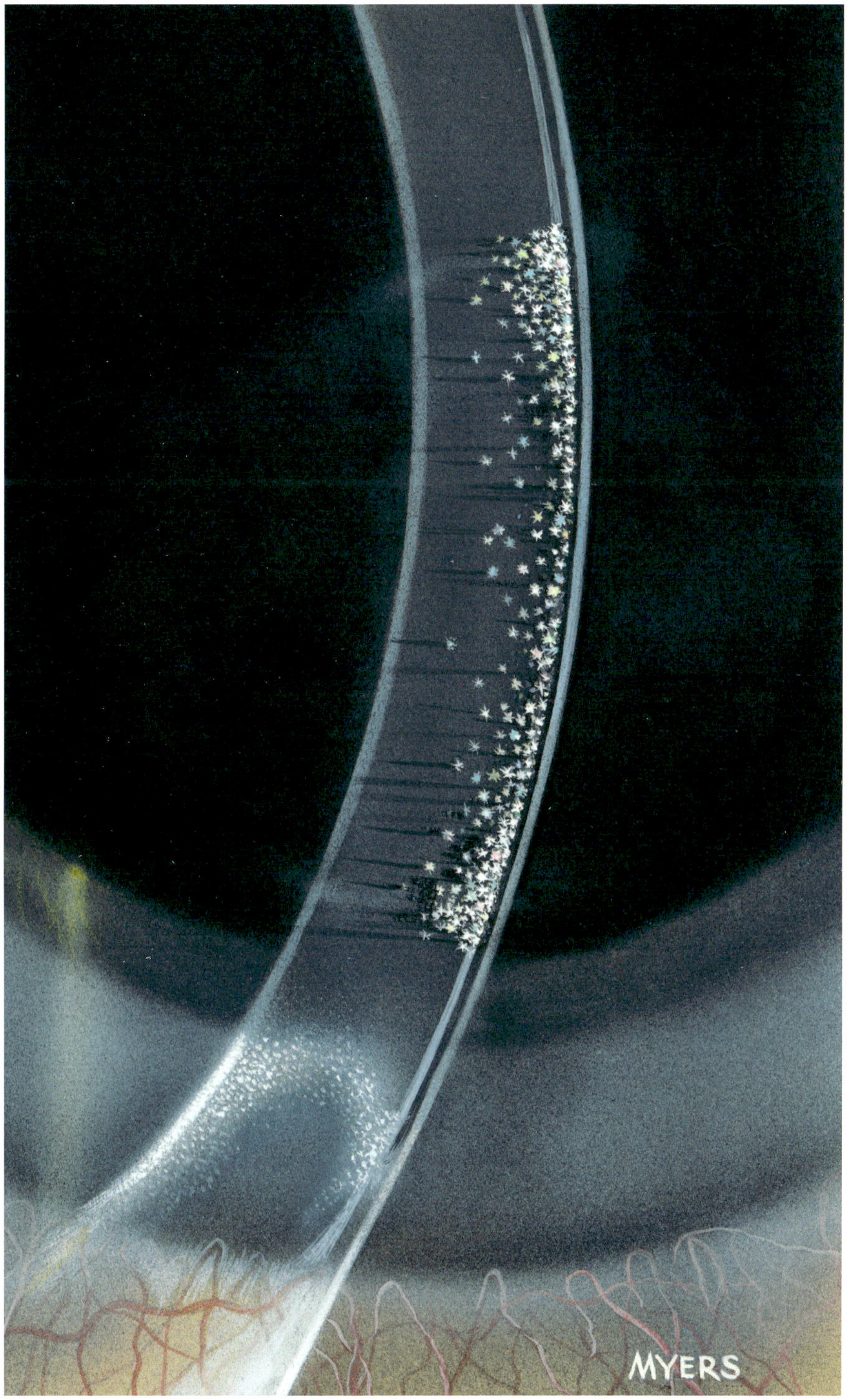
MYERS

PLATES 17 & 18

Granular Corneal Dystrophy

PLATE 17

An autosomal dominant genetically inherited stromal dystrophy, at the 5q31 locus, characterized by white, crumb-like granular deposits. The opacities are discrete and centrally located with clear stroma between the lesions, this often allowing for good vision until the opacities become more confluent. Superficially located deposits are related to recurrent erosions which lead to superficial scarring. In this painting, the deposits are relatively mild, but do extend to the mid-periphery of the cornea. Superiorly, there is an area of corneal opacity unrelated to the dystrophic changes.

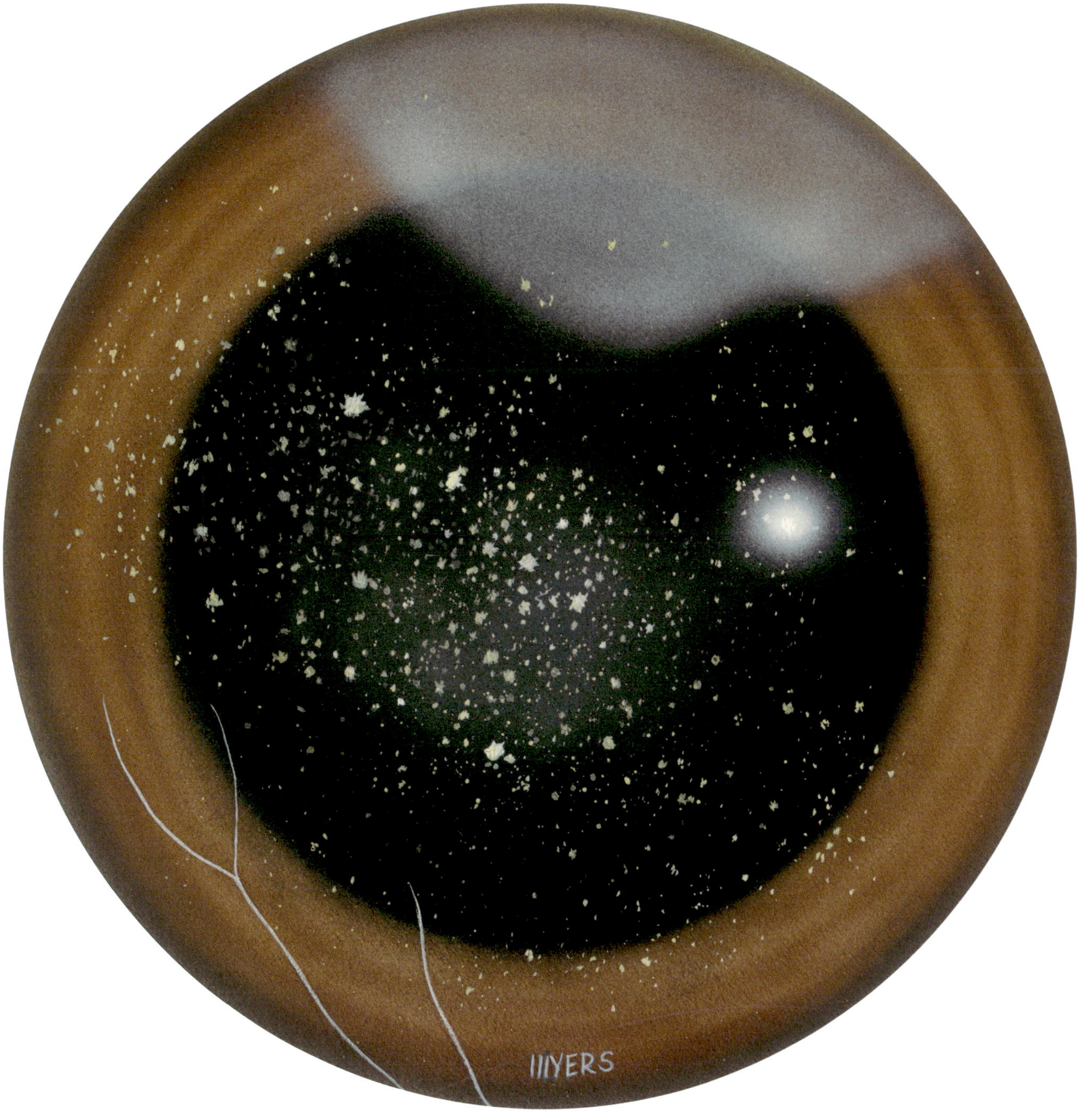
MYERS

PLATE 18

This slit-beam view illustrates the deposition of hyaline material throughout the stroma, although more often in less advanced cases such as this, the deposits are more concentrated in the anterior corneal stroma. Granular Corneal Dystrophy is closely related to both Reis-Bücklers and Thiel-Behnke corneal dystrophies (Plates 10 to 14), and when the granular dystrophic changes are located in the anterior stroma, they may represent a variant of these dystrophies, not surprisingly since all three are genetically similar.

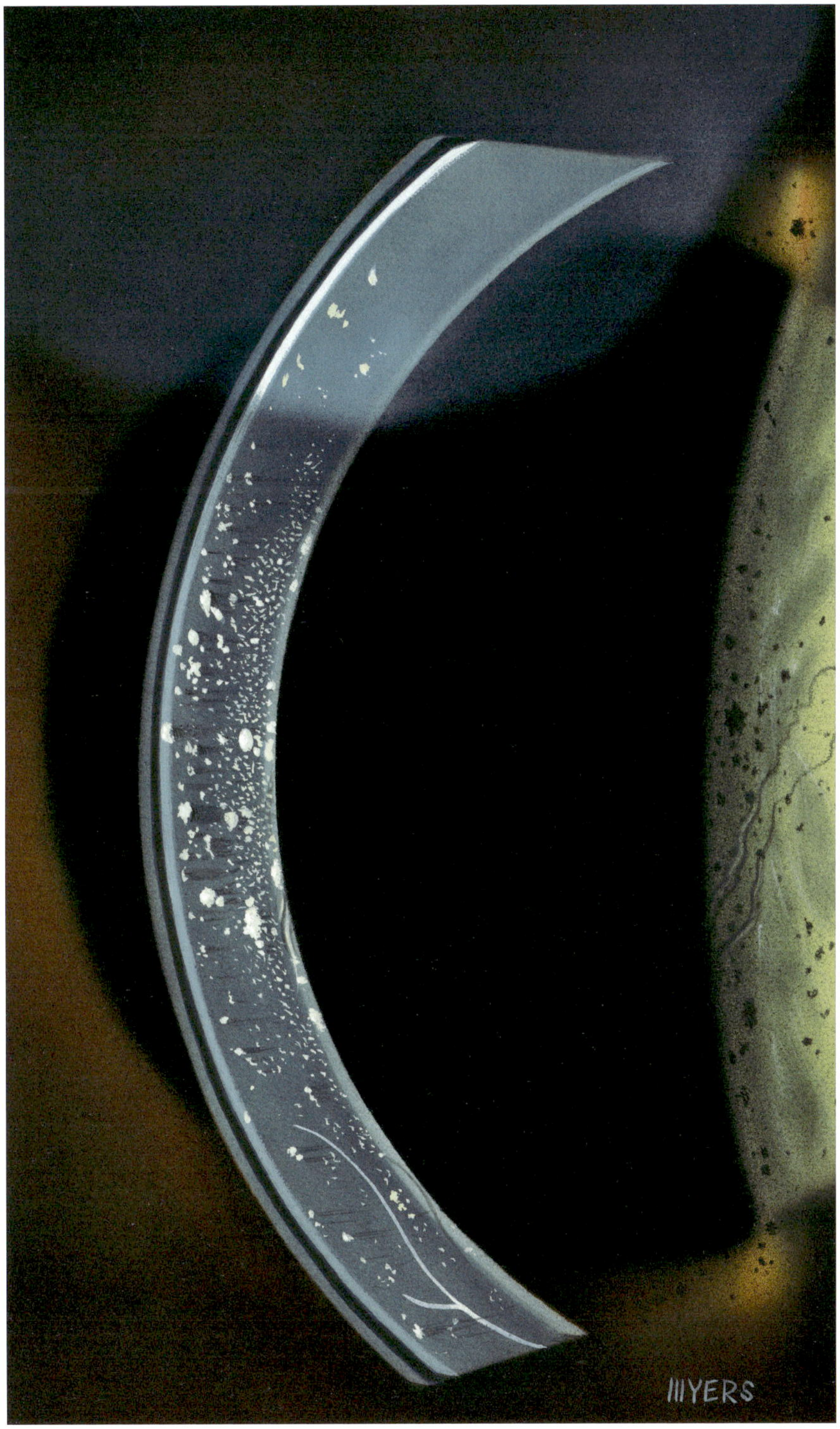
MYERS

PLATES 19 & 20

Granular Corneal Dystrophy

PLATE 19

This painting demonstrates the same dystrophy as in Plates 17 and 18, but in a more advanced stage with a different appearance which is characterized by radiating club-like, denser deposits. Certain pedigrees of familial relationship manifest similar patterns of opacities, while others have only the crumb-like deposits, as seen in Plates 17 and 18.

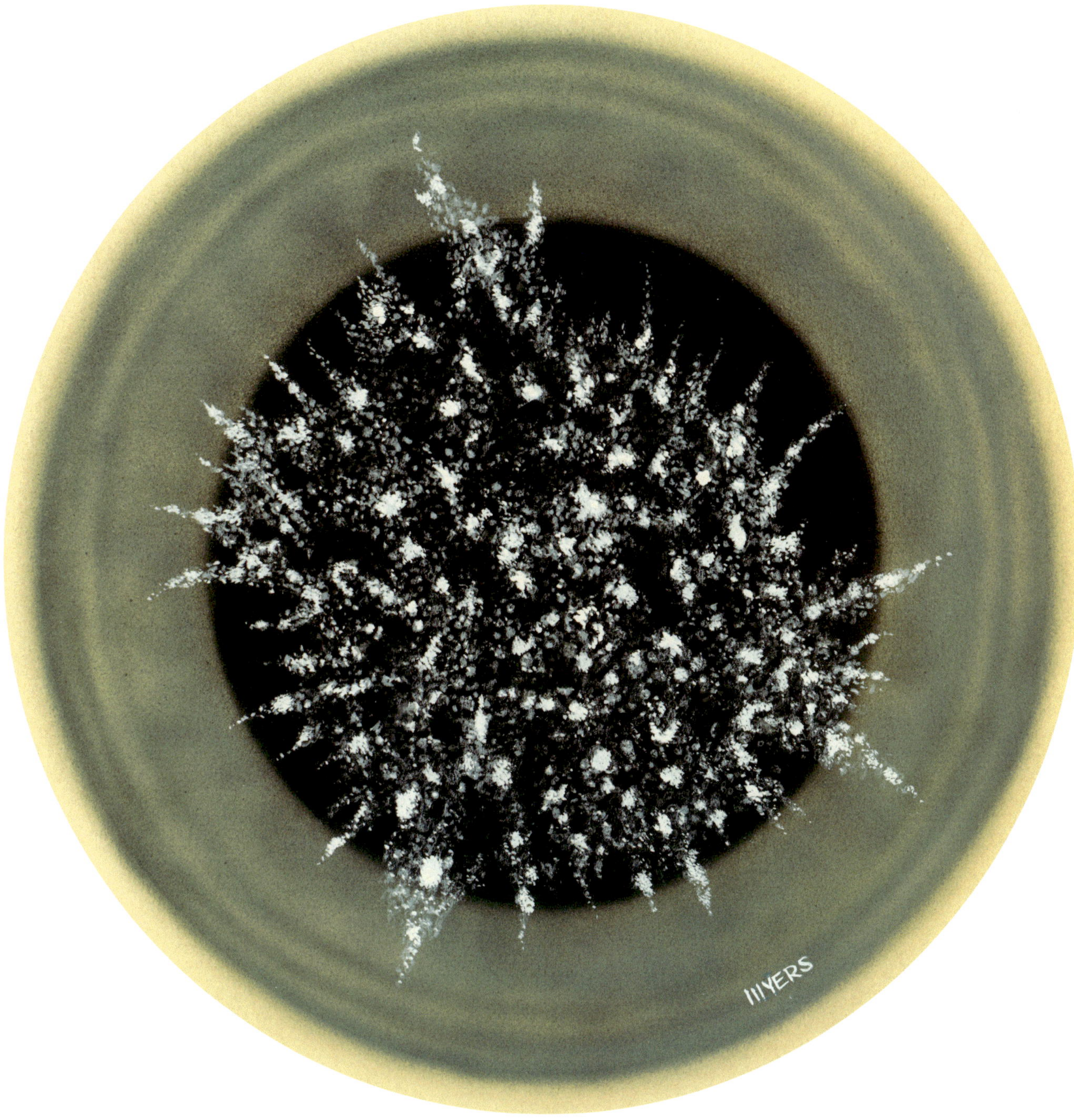
MYERS

PLATE 20

This slit-beam view demonstrates the full-thickness depth of opacities throughout the corneal stroma. In addition, this painting shows a feature that occasionally accompanies this dystrophy in which corneal guttata appear as bleb-like excrescences at the posterior-most layer of the cornea. Although somewhat exaggerated in size, Mr. Myers calls attention to this concomitant finding.

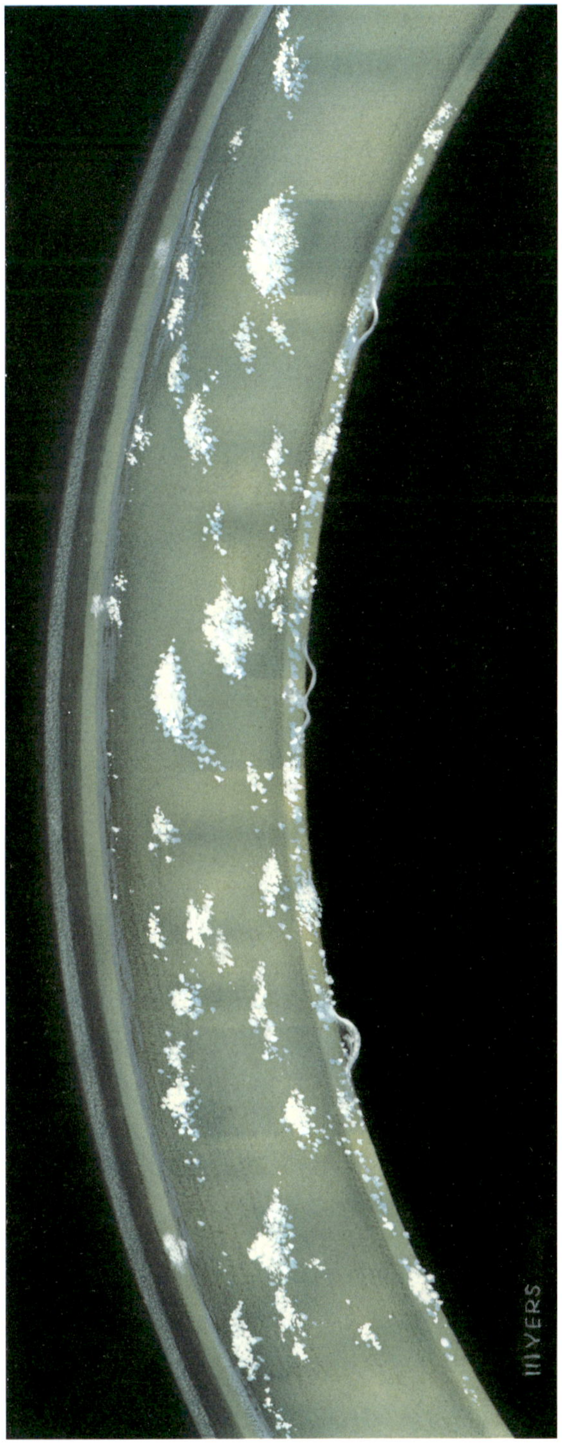

PLATES 21 & 22

Lattice Corneal Dystrophy

PLATE 21

A dominantly inherited corneal dystrophy, genetically similar to Granular Dystrophy (locus5q31), but with a different phenotype or appearance characterized by a branching, refractile linear pattern. Clear corneal stroma between the deposits aids in retention of good vision usually until middle age; however, if the opacities are near the surface of the cornea, they often lead to recurrent erosions with subsequent subepithelial scarring which can reduce vision.

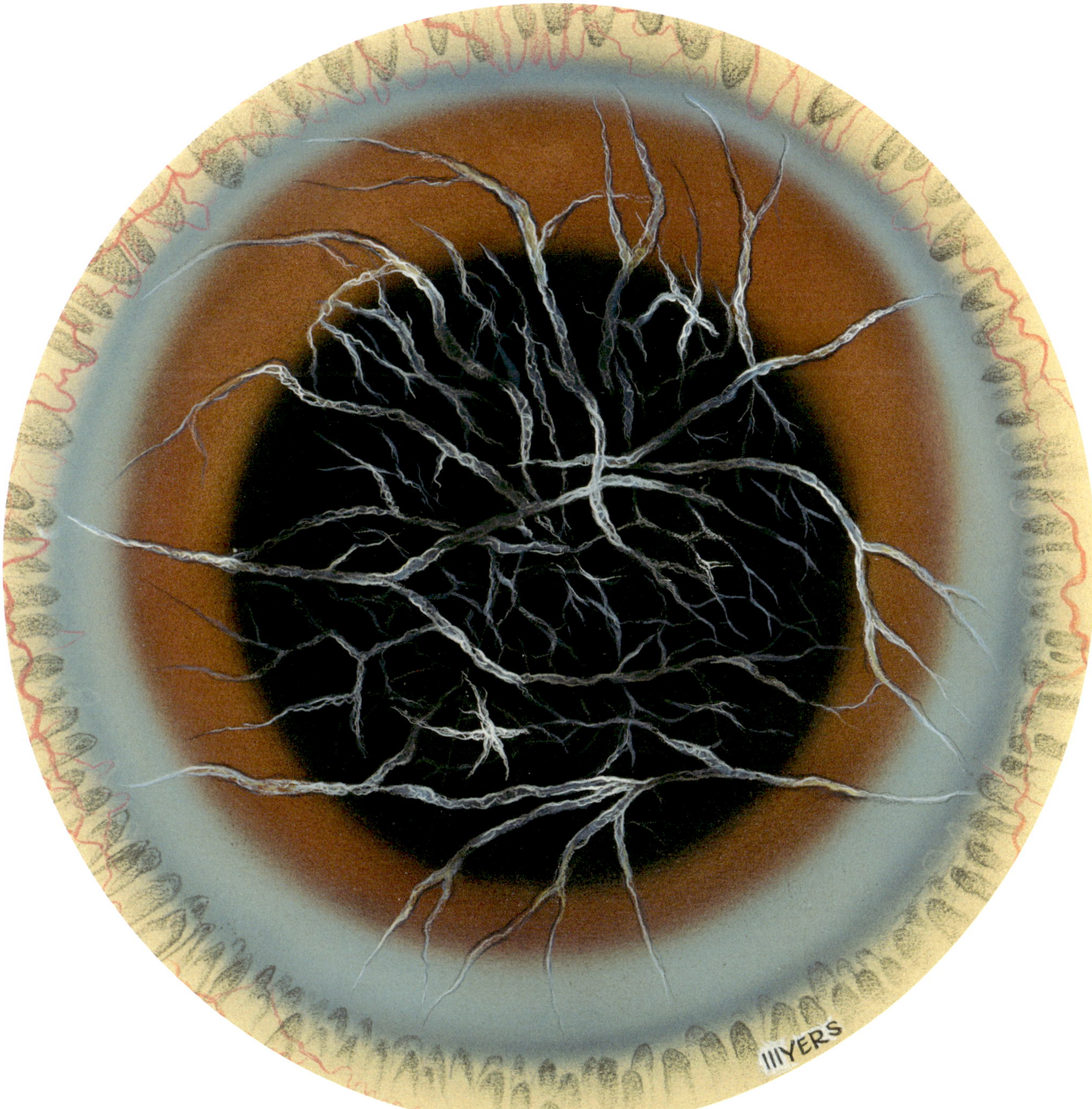
MYERS

PLATE 22

This slit-beam view beautifully captures the refractile lines at varying depths of the corneal stroma, also demonstrating the associated haze around the lines and other more subtle punctate deposits. The refractile, glass-like lines are distinctive for this dystrophy.

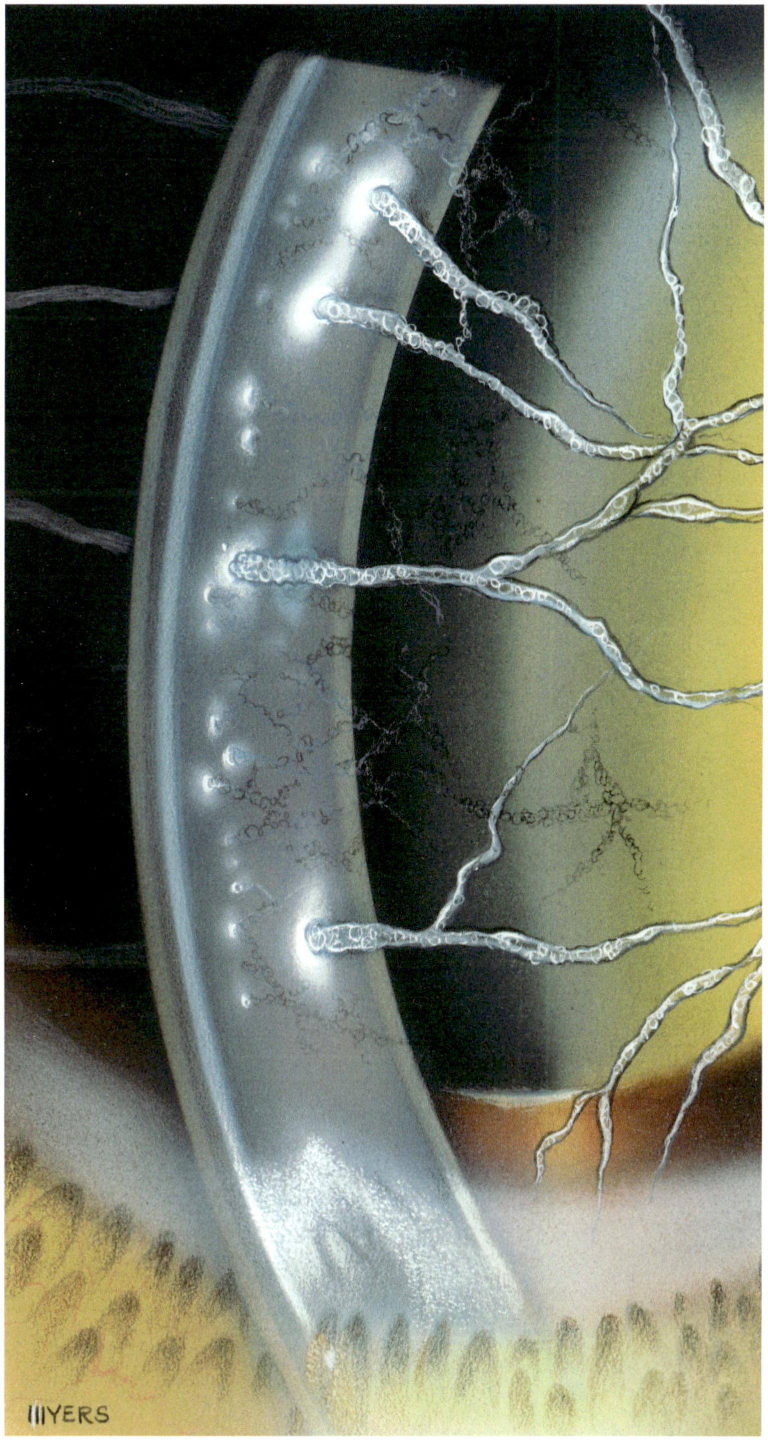
MYERS

PLATES 23 & 24

Lattice Corneal Dystrophy

PLATE 23

The refractile appearance of the linear deposits stand out against the background of a darker iris. The lines consist of a deposit of amyloid material; multiple genotypic variations are characterized by amyloidogenic mutations.

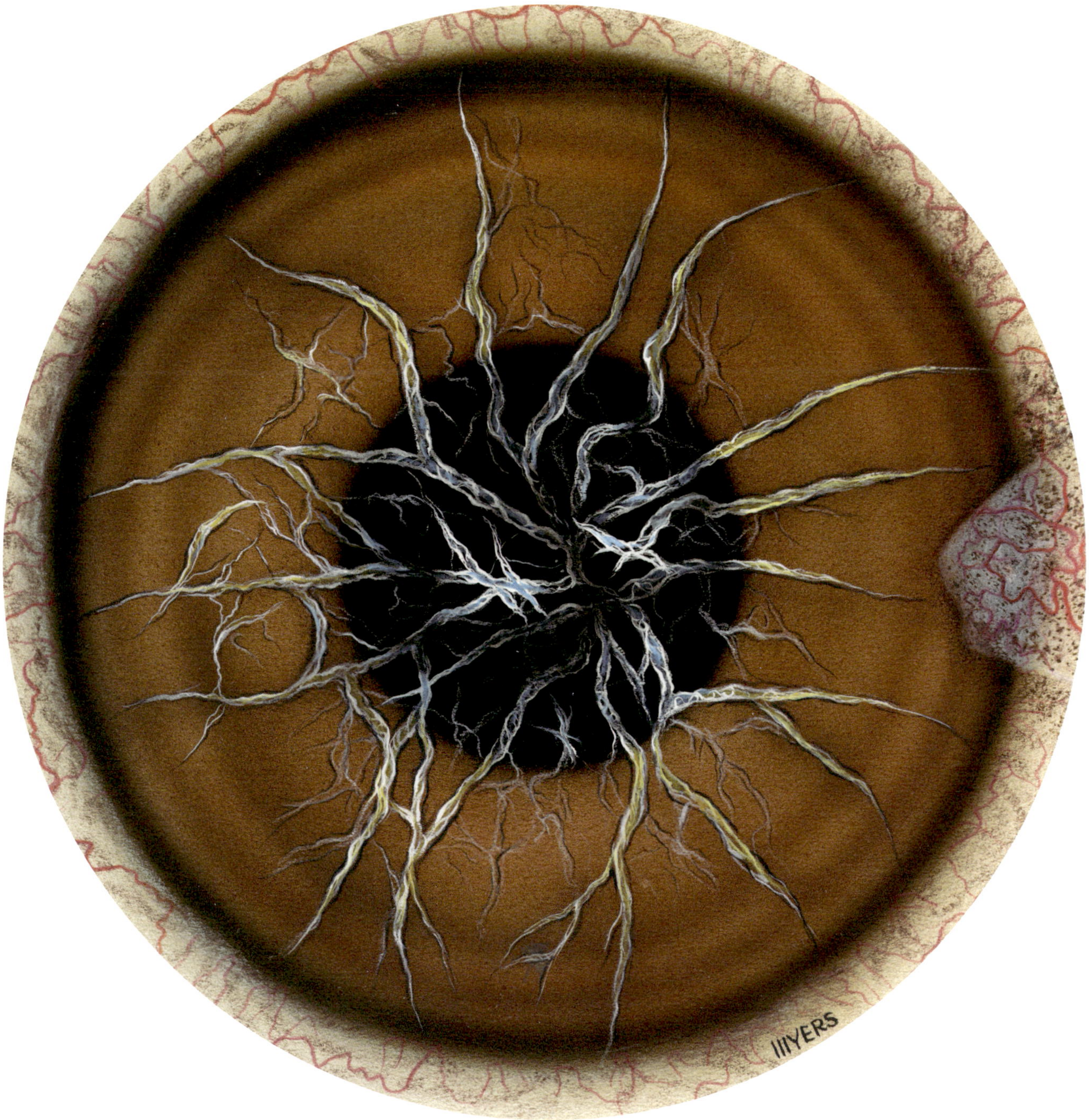
MYERS

PLATE 24

Considerable variability in the location of the linear deposits may lead to symptoms of ocular irritation due to recurrent epithelial erosions. I have noted a distinct correlation between the location of the epithelial erosions in this entity and the proximity of the deposits to the subepithelial surface. The superficial location is especially well-demonstrated in this slit-beam view, which is not appreciated more centrally against the partial transillumination of the iris background.

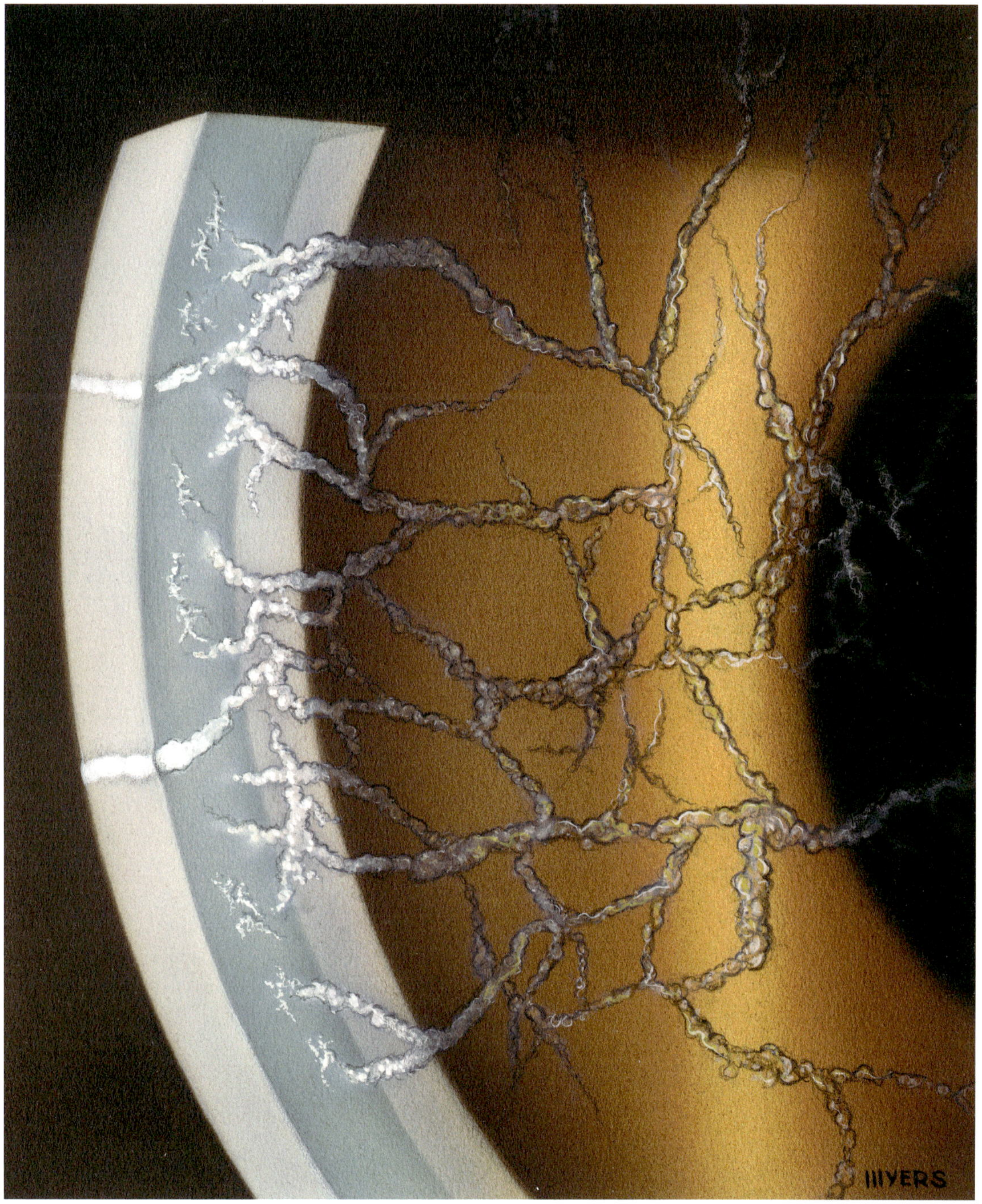
MYERS

PLATES 25 & 26

Macular Corneal Dystrophy

PLATE 25

An autosomal recessive inherited corneal dystrophy characterized by superficial large gray opacities overlying a diffuse corneal haze. The opacities consist of glycosaminoglycan accumulation and typically progress slowly, but affect vision at an early age, in the second to fourth decade, due to the diffuse corneal haze and irritation from the slightly elevated corneal lesions and surface erosions.

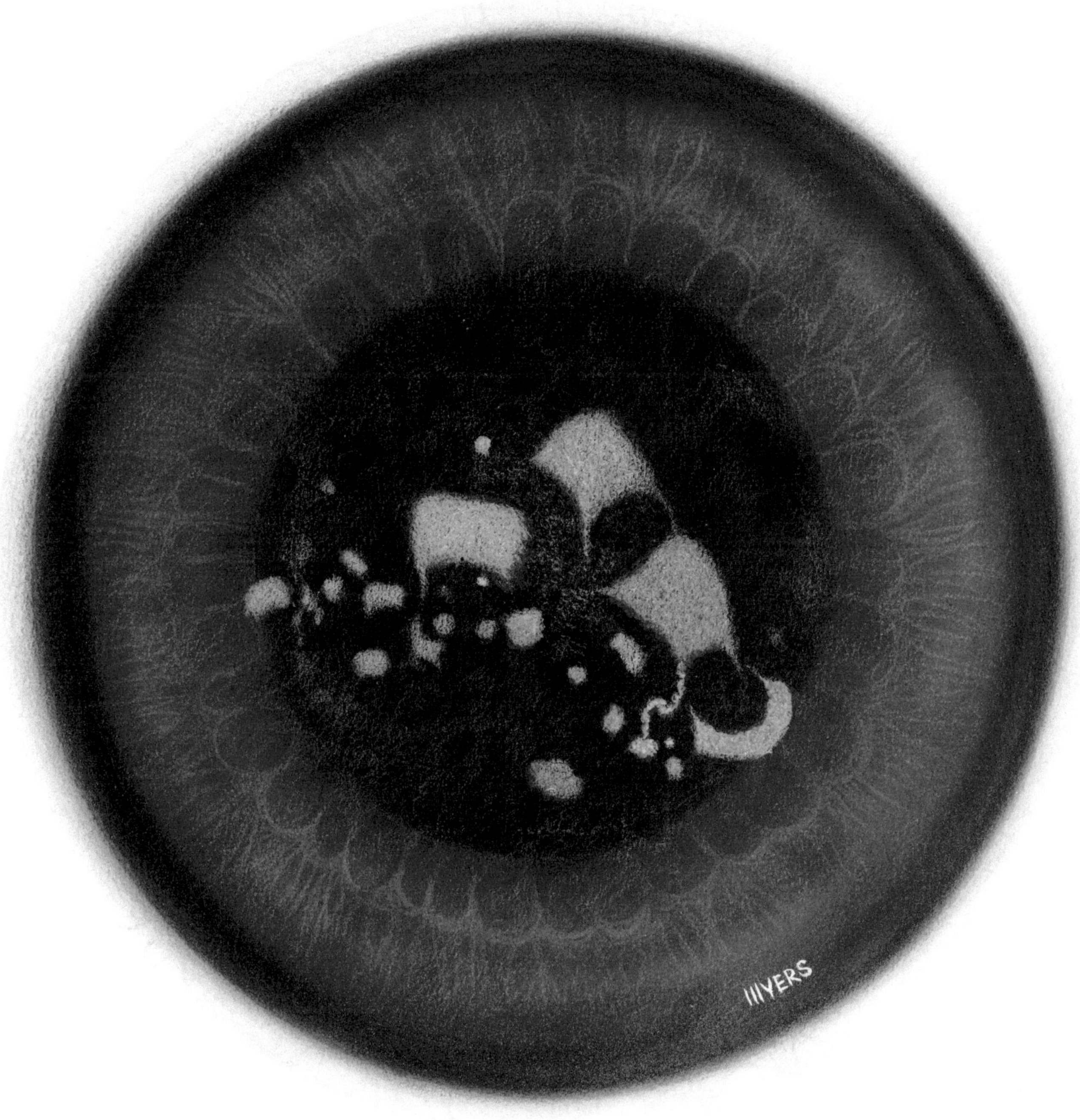

PLATE 26

This slit-beam view demonstrates the superficial, somewhat elevated, location of the maculae. This accounts for the severe visual impairment and photophobia experienced by patients affected with this entity. In addition, the diffuse stromal haze is well depicted throughout the cornea. Unlike granular and lattice dystrophies, there are no clear areas between the deposits, therefore resulting in earlier visual impairment and the need for keratoplasty. Because of the recessive inheritance pattern, it is more common than granular and lattice dystrophies in areas of the world with high rates of consanguinity.

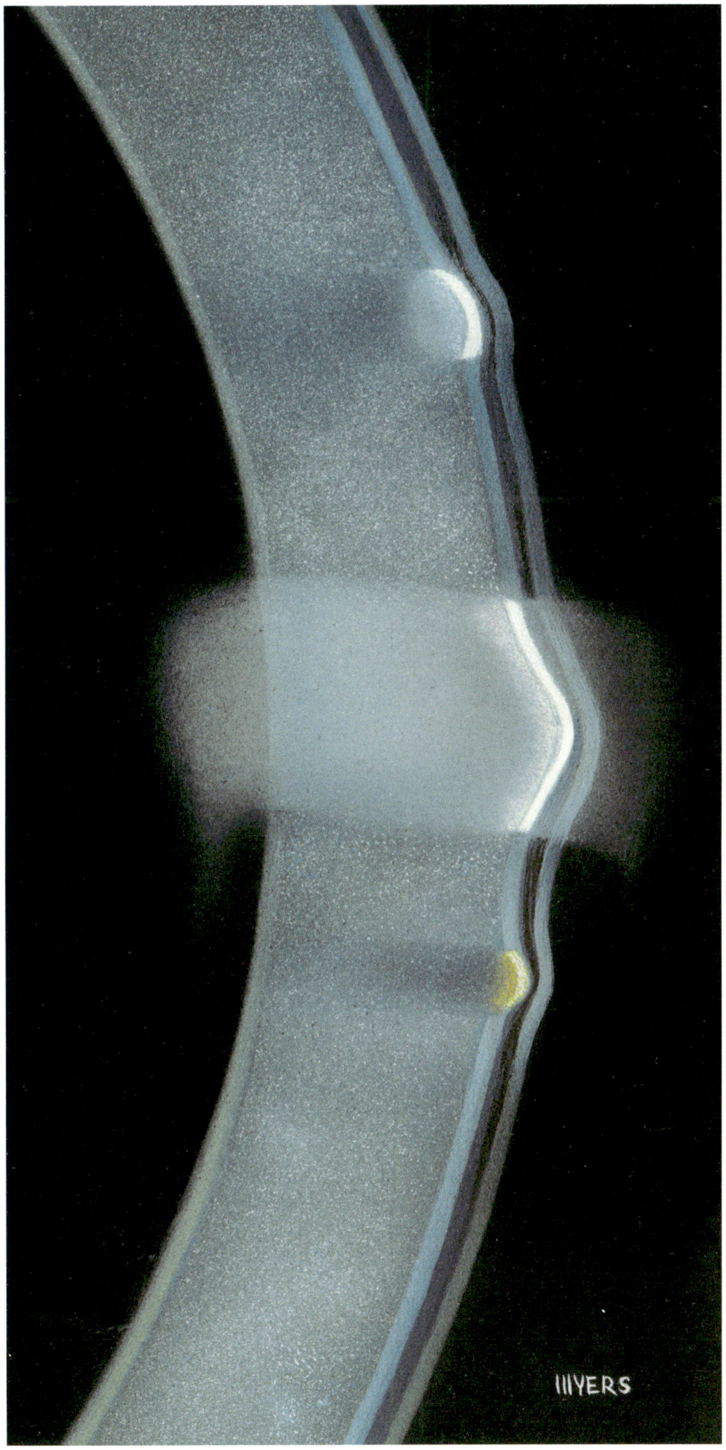
MYERS

PLATES 27 & 28

Fleck Corneal Dystrophy

PLATE 27

Previously referred to as François-Neetens Speckled Corneal Dystrophy, this is an autosomal dominant inherited stromal dystrophy characterized by tiny, discrete, flat and wreath-like or ring-shaped subtle gray opacities scattered in the corneal stroma. Since it is asymptomatic, causing no visual impairment and only recognized incidentally on corneal examination with biomicroscopic magnification, it is seldom recognized.

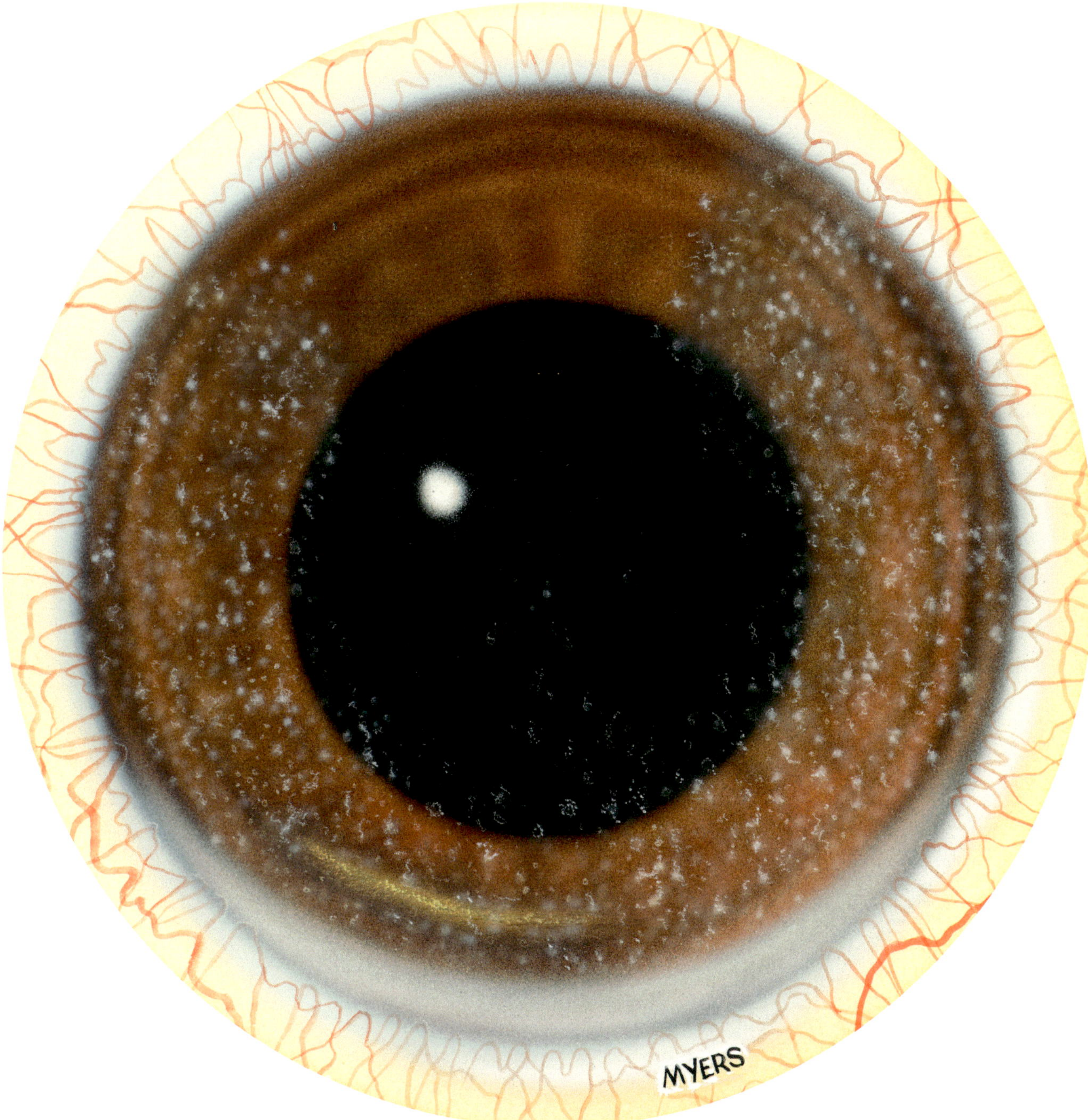
MYERS

PLATE 28

The slit-beam view emphasizes the location of the lesions throughout the corneal stroma, even approaching the corneal periphery. However, either this patient had a most unusual number of deposits, or Mr. Myers exaggerated the number of lesions to characterize the location and diffuse distribution. Usually the lesions are very sparse and overlooked. The opacities represent swollen stromal keratocytes with intracellular deposition of glycosaminoglycans and lipid.

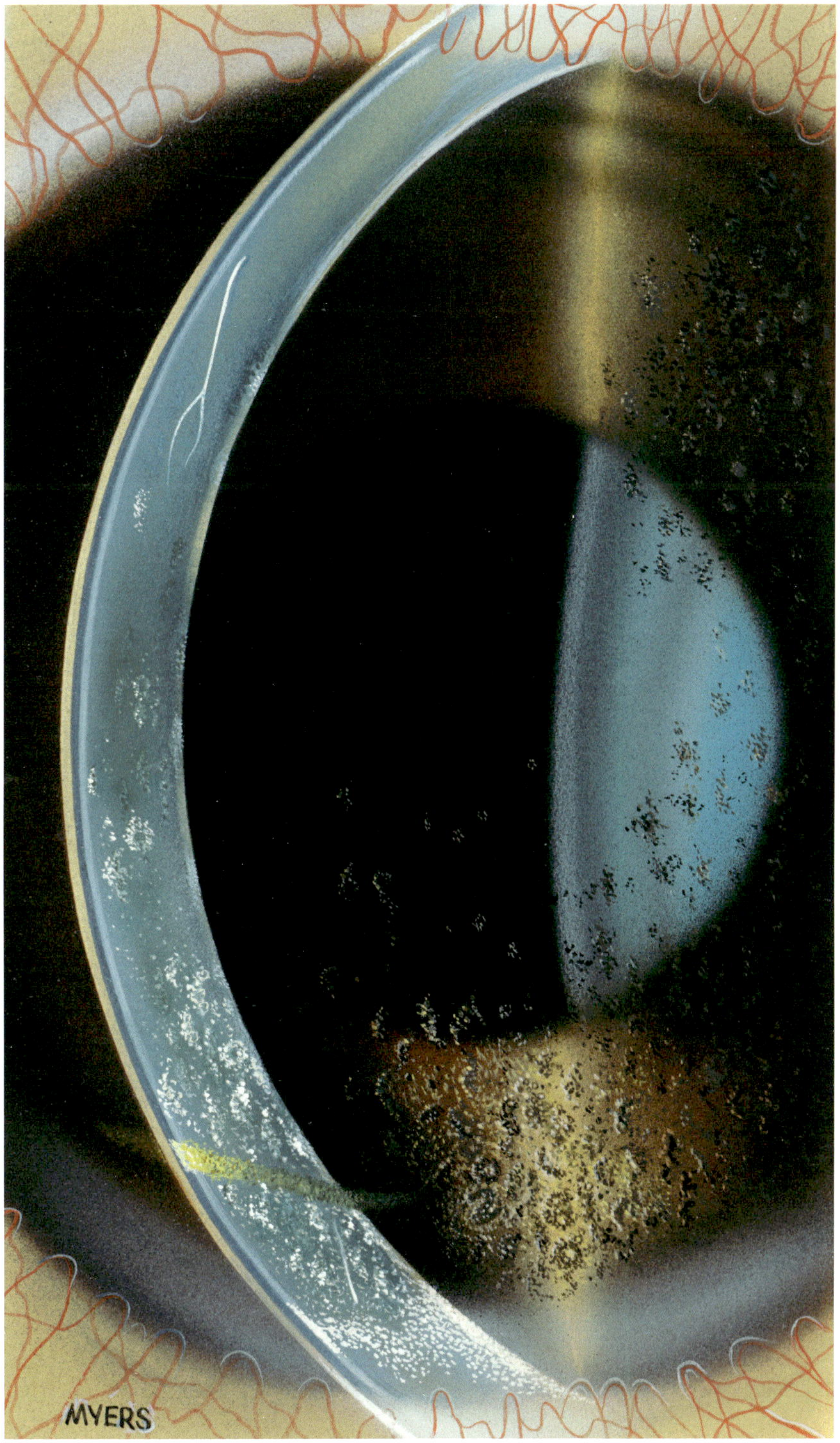
MYERS

PLATES 29 & 30

Central Cloudy Dystrophy of François

A not uncommon deep corneal pattern of opacity that has been classified as a dystrophy, but with unknown inheritance.

PLATE 29

The changes are characterized by a pattern of posterior "crocodile-shagreen," with soft gray tile-like polygonal opacities surrounded by clear grout-like lines. A similar pattern is commonly recognized as a peripheral corneal aging change in older patients, but without central involvement. Histologically, the lesions have been shown to contain acid-mucopolysaccarides.

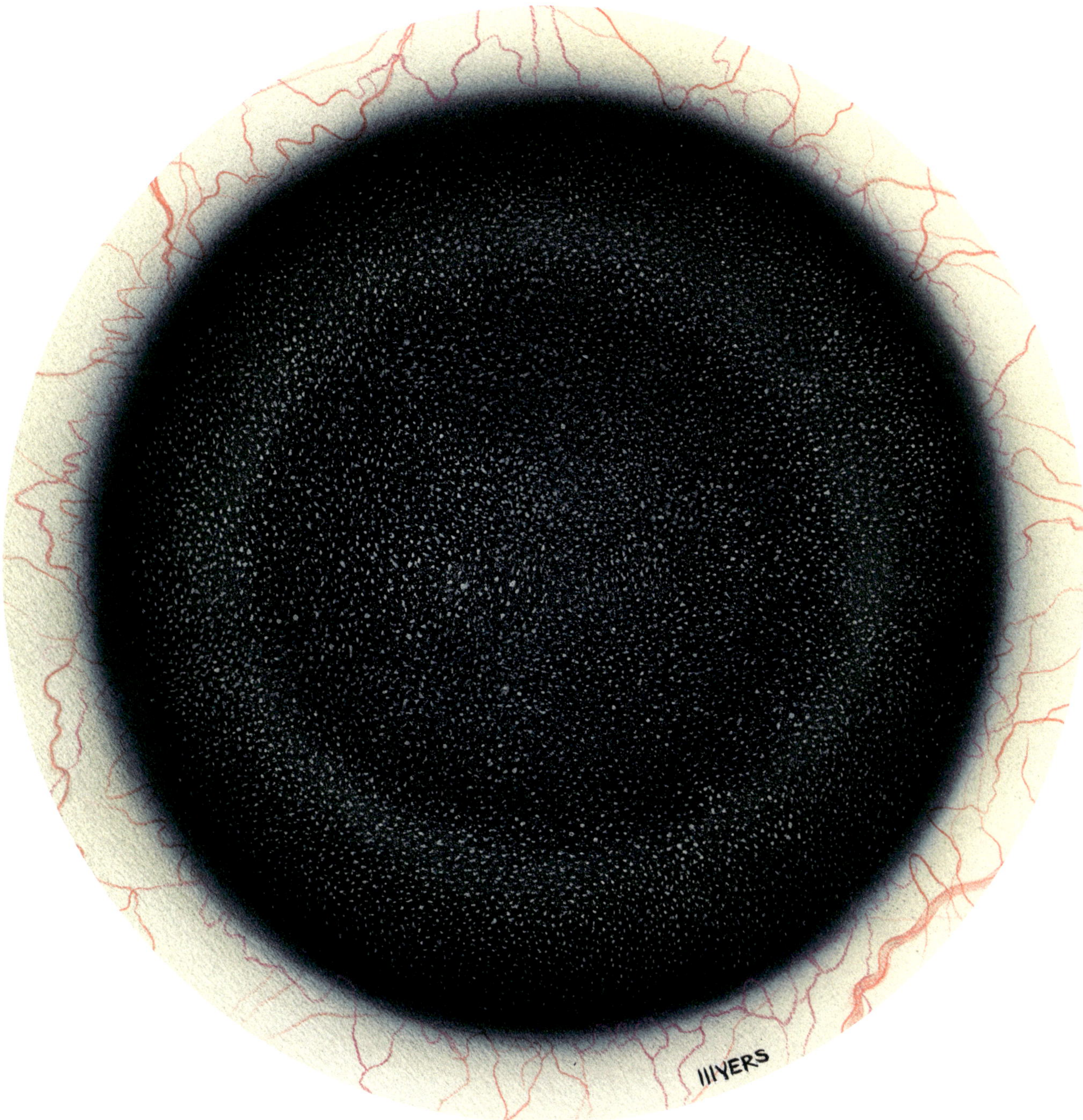
IIIYERS

PLATE 30

At the risk of being presumptuous, I think Mr. Myers did not fully recognize the features of these deep changes. He depicted the lesions as small, without the hallmark and typical "tile-like" appearance. On the other hand, he does demonstrate the clear areas surrounding the lesions. He probably overlooked the configuration of these deposits and confirmed the adage that "we see what we know, but do not see what we don't know."

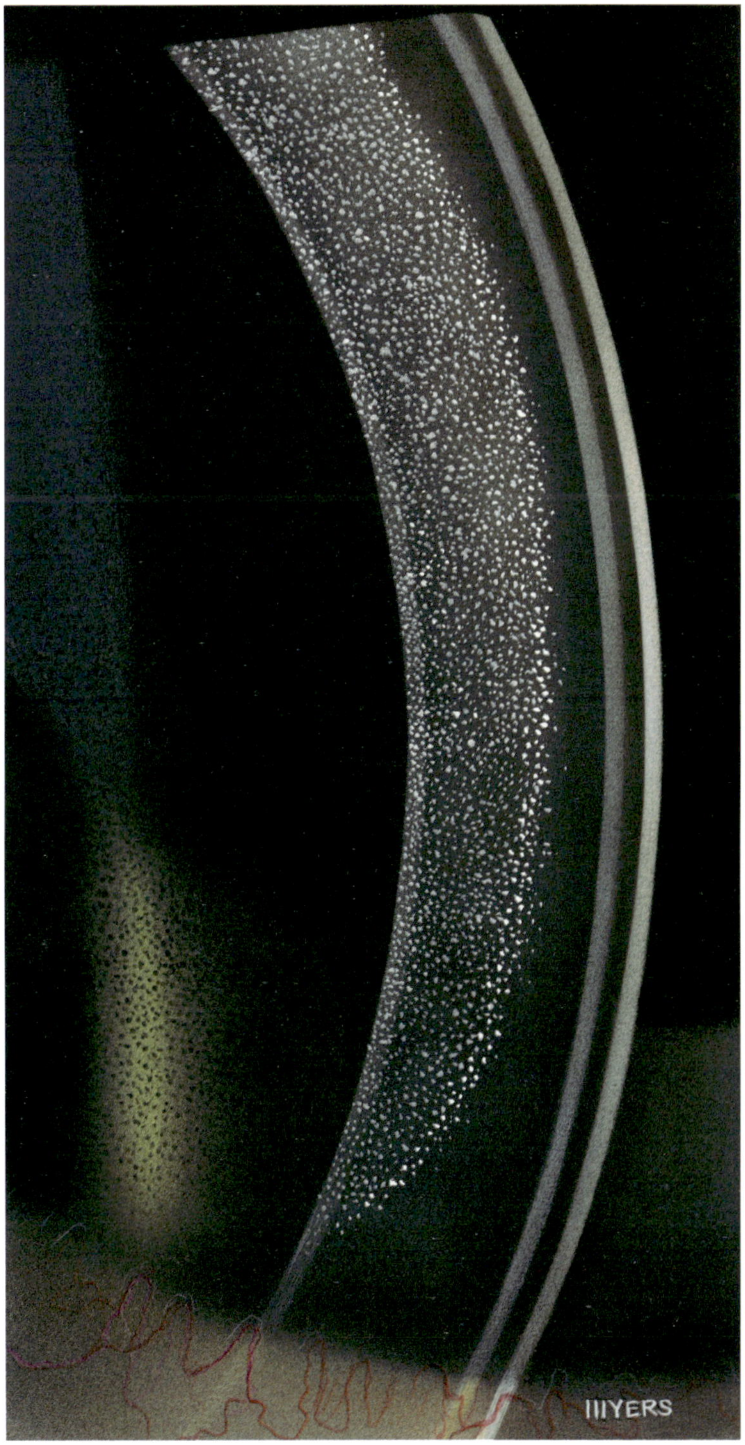
MYERS

PLATES 31 & 32

Posterior Polymorphous Corneal Dystrophy

This autosomal dominant dystrophy, with occasional unilateral presentation without apparent heredity, is characterized by posterior polymorphous corneal lesions of varying shapes, with deep corneal vacuoles often in a curvilinear "snail-tract"-like pattern. In contrast to most other corneal dystrophies which tend to have involvement in the central cornea and are usually symmetrical, the polymorphous deep corneal appearance in this dystrophy tends to be asymmetrical and often involves only the mid-periphery.

PLATE 31

This painting illustrates the nodular vesicles as either isolated or in clusters with minimal surrounding opacities.

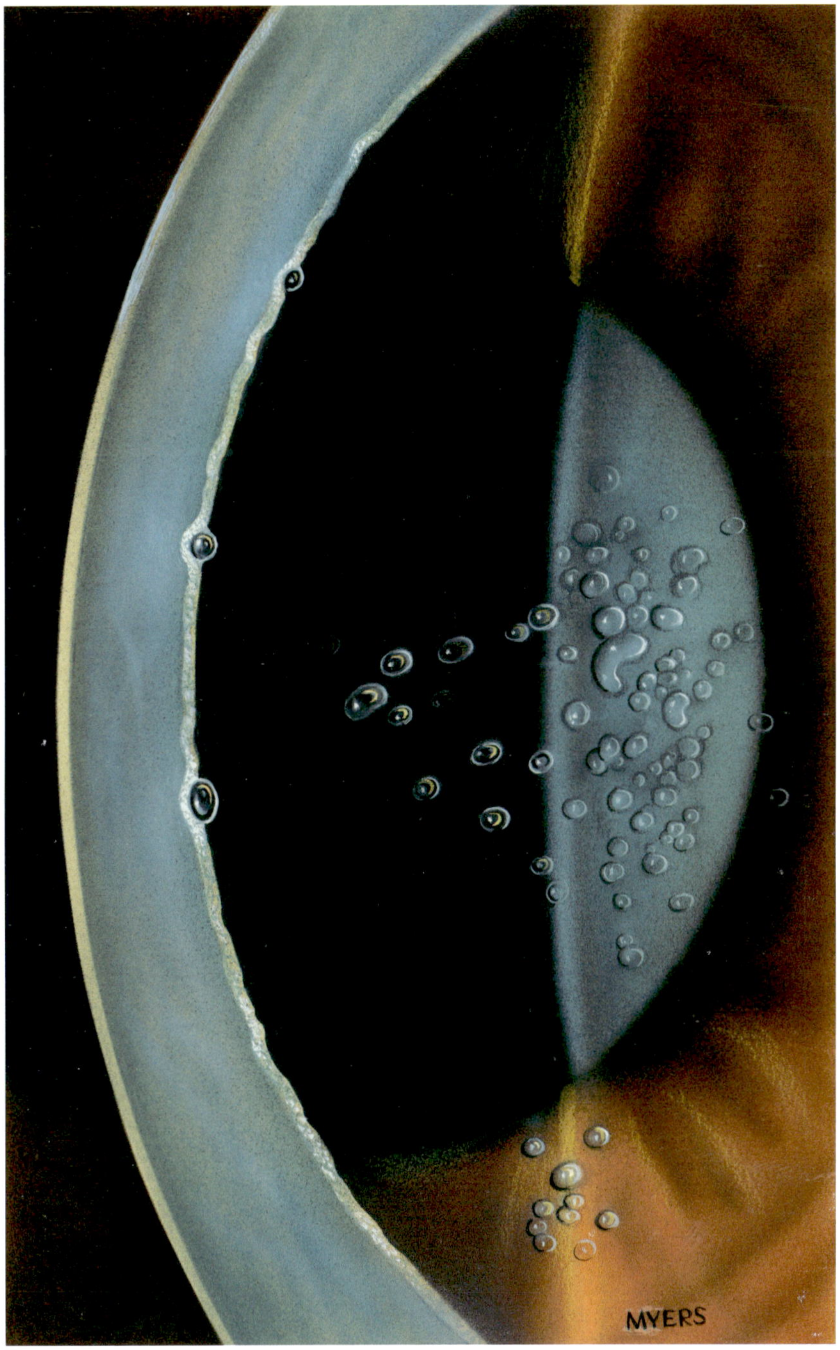
MYERS

PLATE 32

In this illustration, an area of confluent vesicles and surrounding opacity frames the vesicles or tracts, and can lead to endothelial dysfunction and edema. However, in most cases the entity does not progress significantly and does not lead to visual impairment. This dystrophy can be confused with Iridocorneal Endothelial (ICE) syndrome, which is characterized by unilateral diffuse "beaten-metal" endothelial changes associated with iridocorneal adhesions, iris atrophy and membranes, and glaucoma.

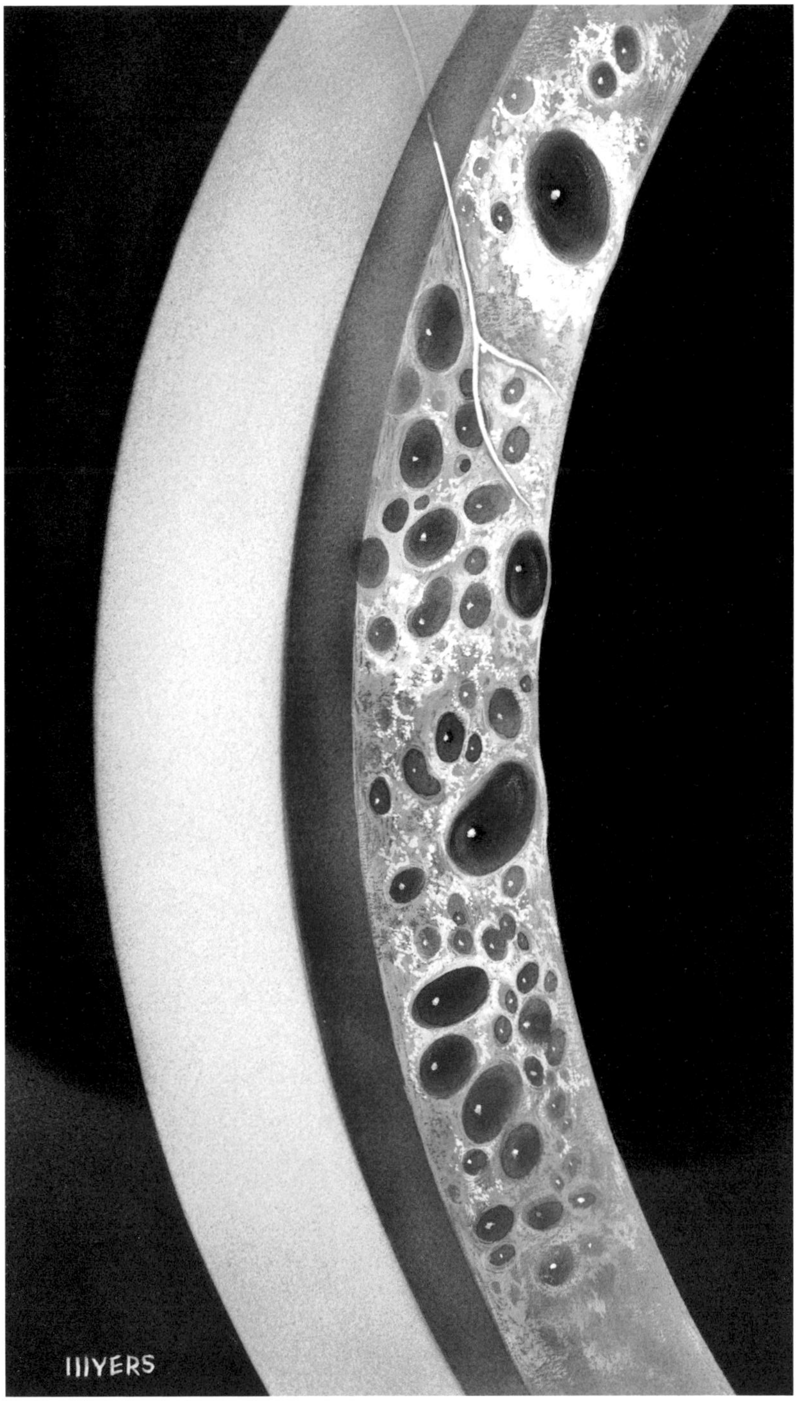
MYERS

PLATES 33 & 34

Cornea Farinata

A rarely recognized pre-Descemet localized corneal degeneration or aging change characterized by flour or grain-like powdery punctuate opacities.

PLATE 33

Combined slit-beam and partial retroillumination view demonstrating the diffusely homogeneous deep corneal opacities. This is an excellent demonstration of the fine punctuate opacities as seen with slit-lamp biomicroscopy. Histopathology has demonstrated intracellular vacuoles containing lipofuscin-like material in posterior stromal keratocytes.

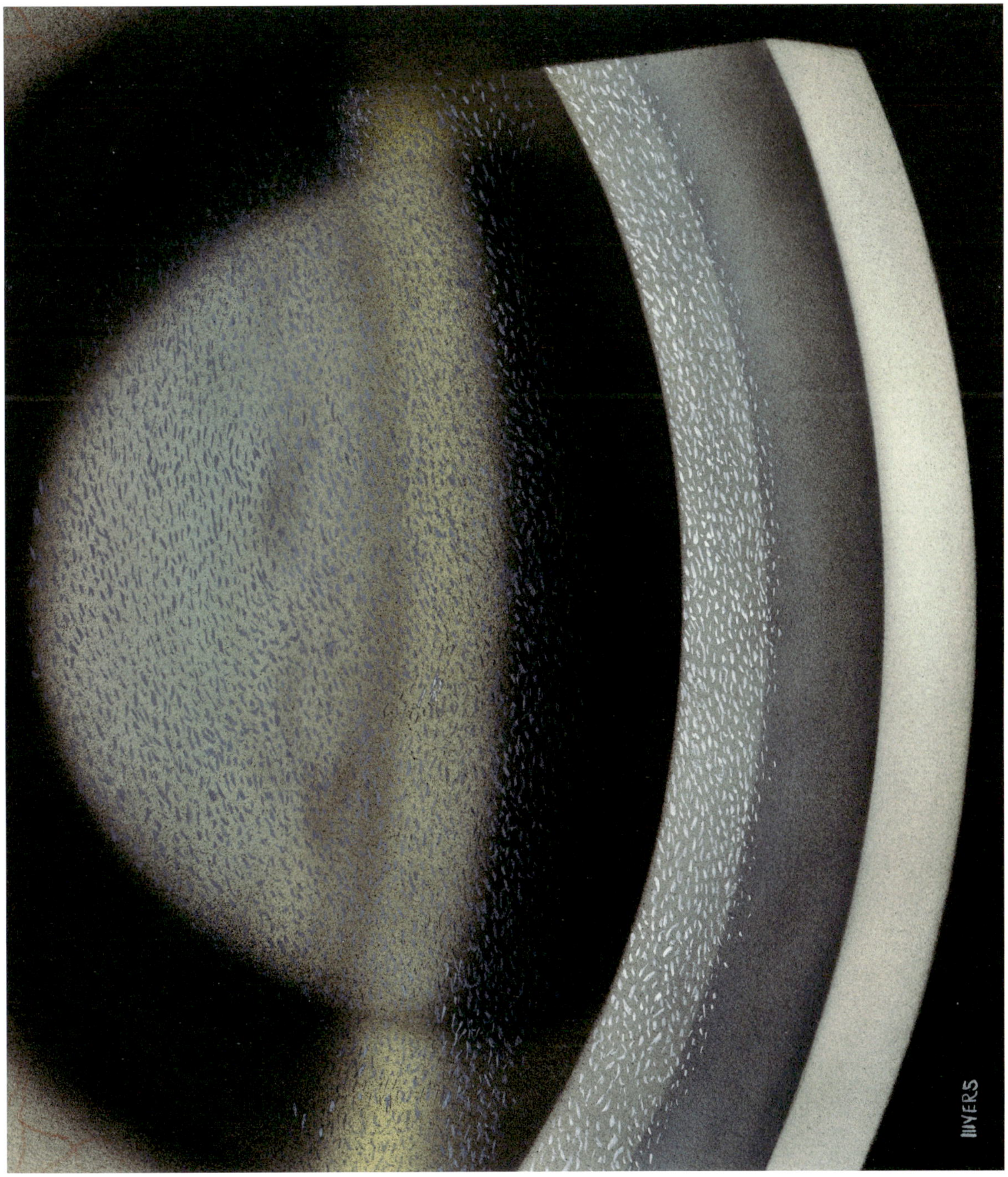
MYERS

PLATE 34

A slit-beam illustration localizing the farina-shaped opacities to the pre-Descemet membrane level in the deep corneal stroma. Note the clear overlying stroma which accounts for insignificant visual impairment.

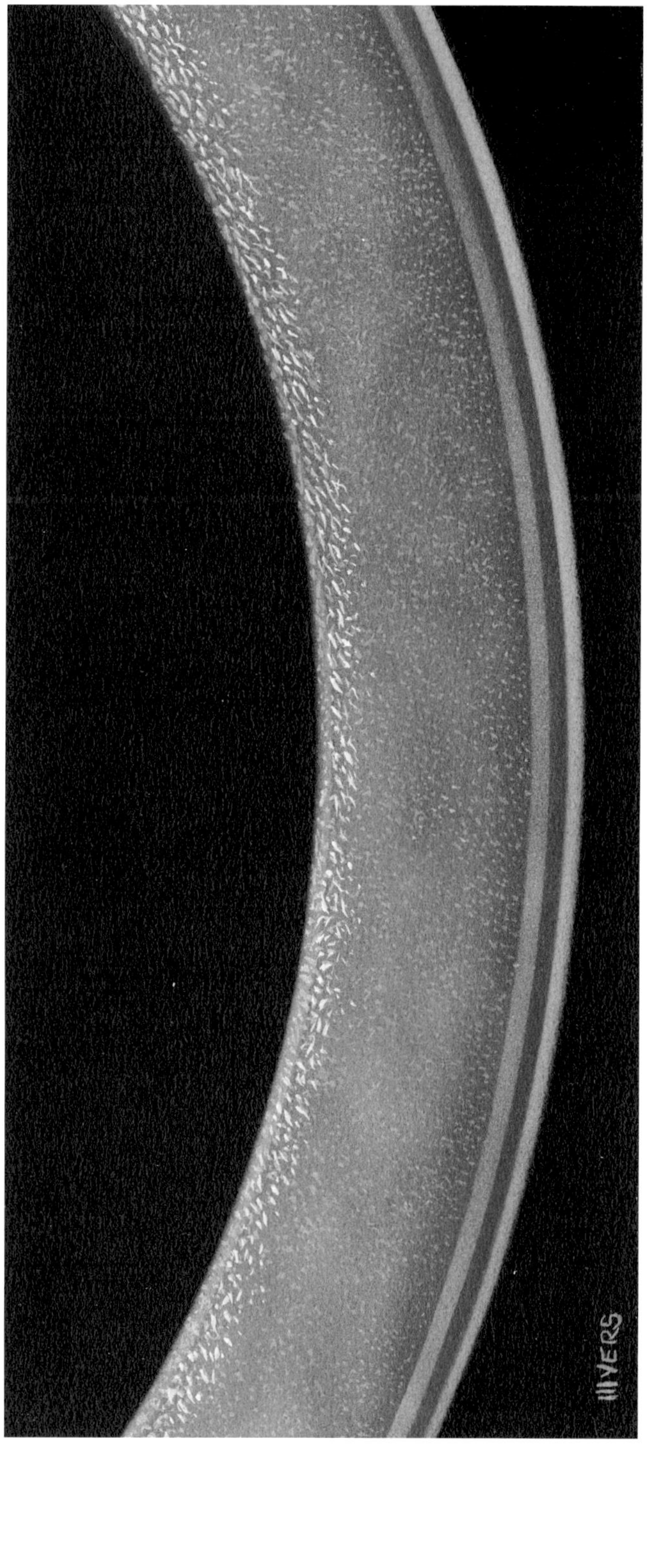

PLATES 35 & 36

Hassall-Henle Bodies of the Peripheral Cornea

These small excrescences of the deep peripheral cornea represent an aging change of the basement membrane of the corneal endothelium. By specular reflection and scleral scatter, they appear as dark circular spots or spaces, larger than individual endothelial cells, and are similar to cornea guttata as seen centrally in Fuchs dystrophy.

PLATE 35

These peripheral changes are localized by Mr. Myers to the inferior and superior cornea, although they can be visualized throughout the corneal periphery. The painting was described as "Lacy Dystrophy."

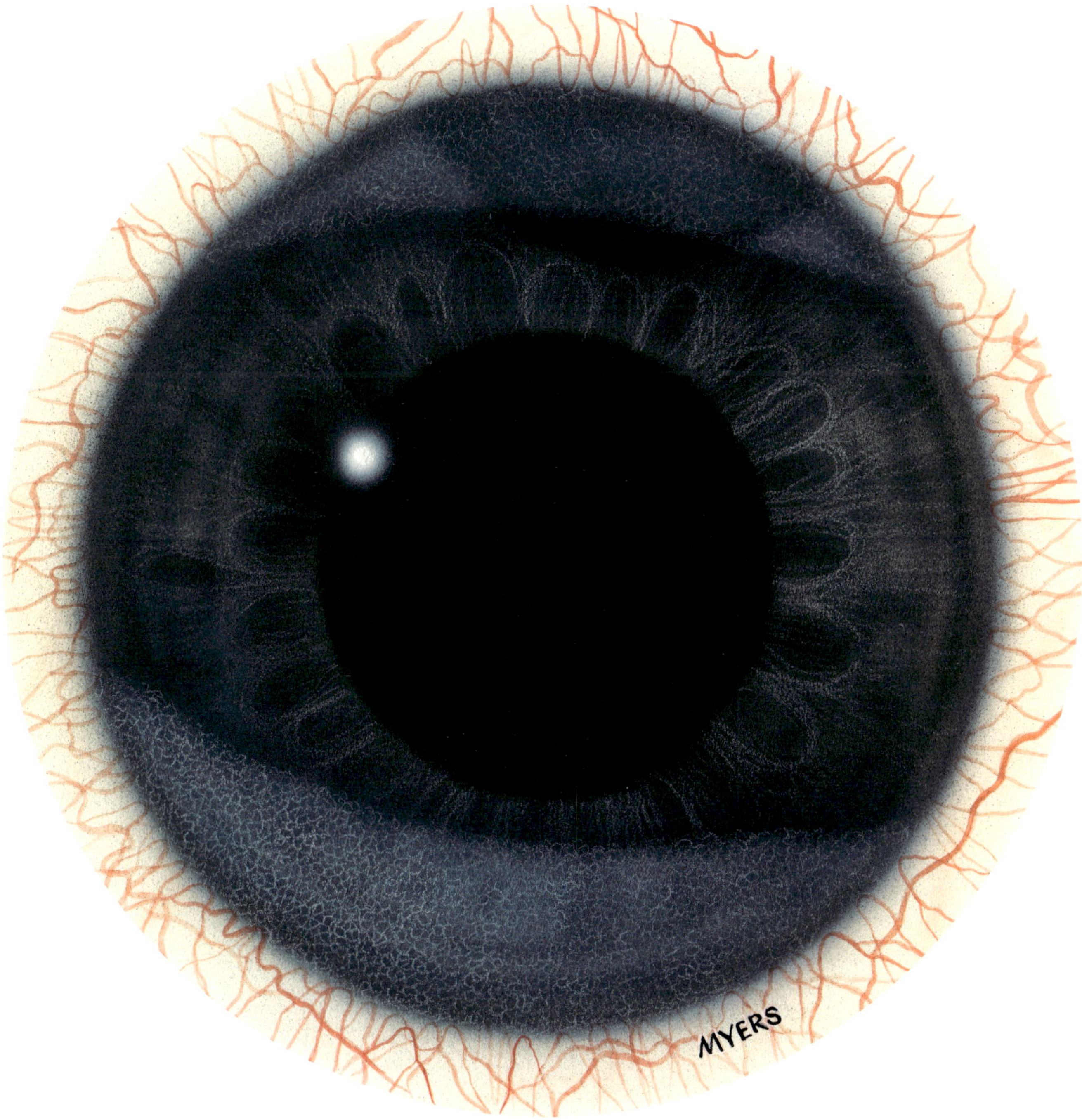
MYERS

PLATE 36

The posterior pattern of peripheral endothelial vacuoles or guttata are beautifully represented as having a lacy border on direct illumination and by dark borders and light vacuoles by retroillumination. Rarely, these abnormal endothelial cells may decompensate resulting in peripheral edema.

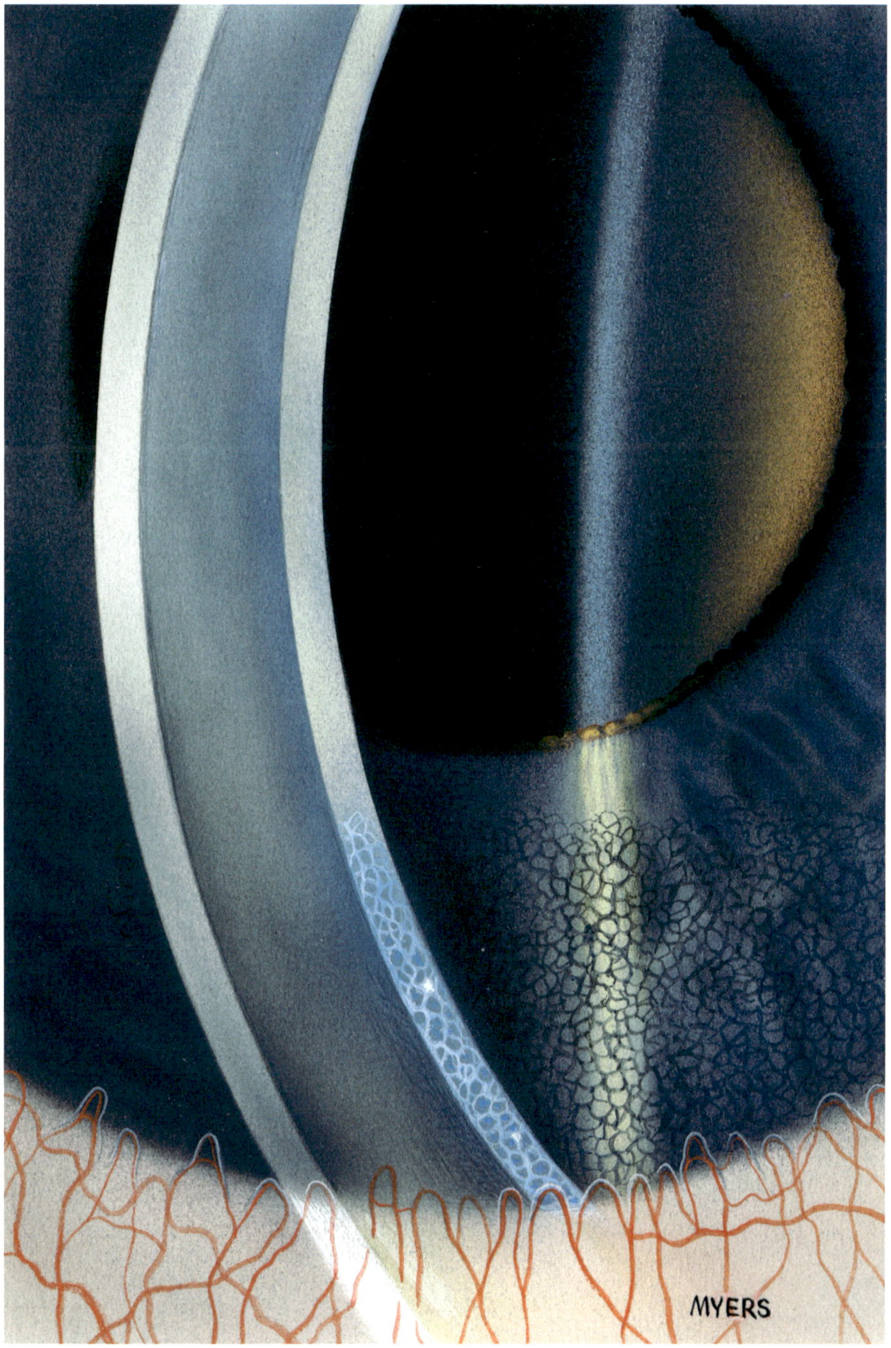
MYERS

PLATES 37 & 38

Corneal Chrysiasis

Corneal deposition of gold is associated with systemic gold therapy used in the treatment of rheumatoid arthritis. As with other heavy metal corneal deposition, gold preferentially deposits in the peripheral deep cornea at the level of Descemet membrane, presumably by diffusion from the perilimbal circulation. Some deposition may also enter the cornea via the aqueous fluid in the anterior chamber or deposit superficially from gold in the tear film. These deposits are of no visual significance, are probably dose- and time-related, and may be partially reversible with cessation of gold therapy.

PLATE 37

This painting demonstrates advanced gold deposition in the deep peripheral cornea. Note that there appears to be some gold-like deposits in the surface subepithelium.

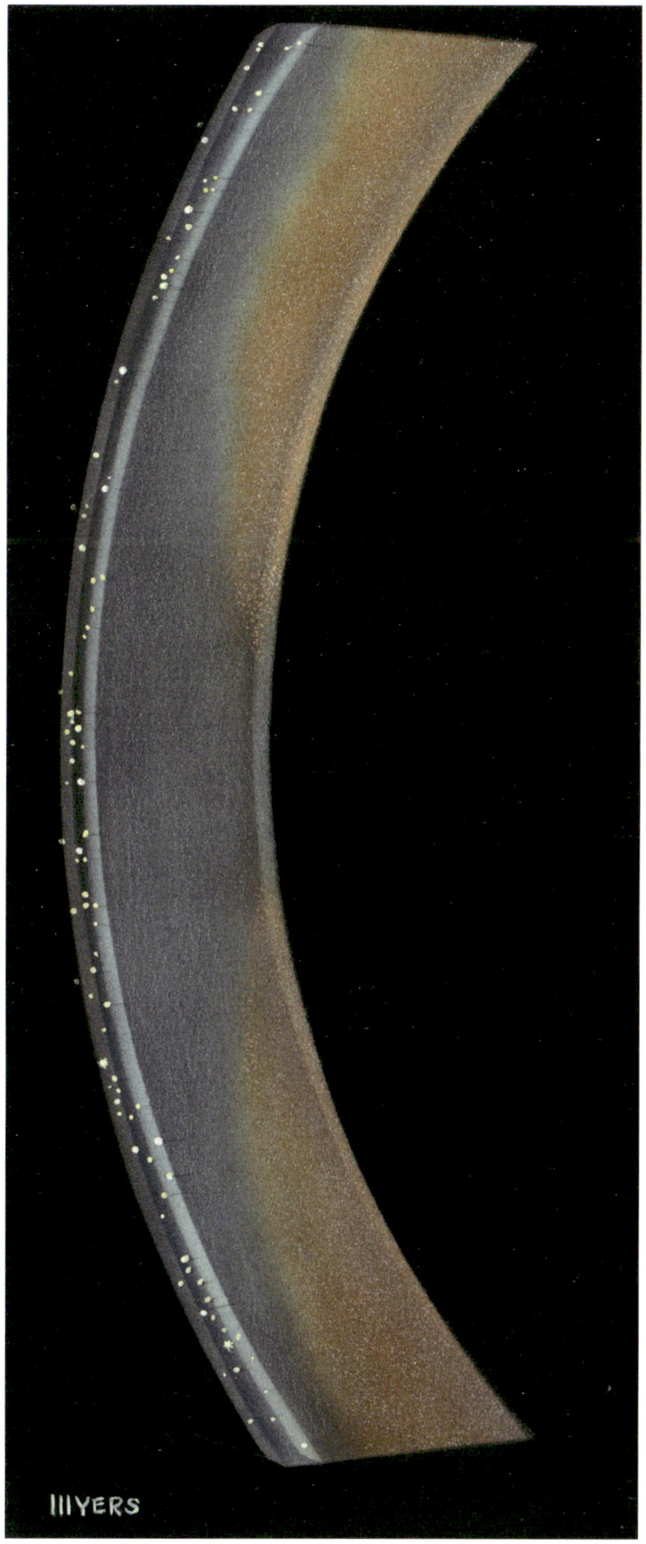
MYERS

PLATE 38

In this illustration, a lesser degree of gold deposition is located along Descemet membrane posteriorly and also at the corneal subepithelial level.

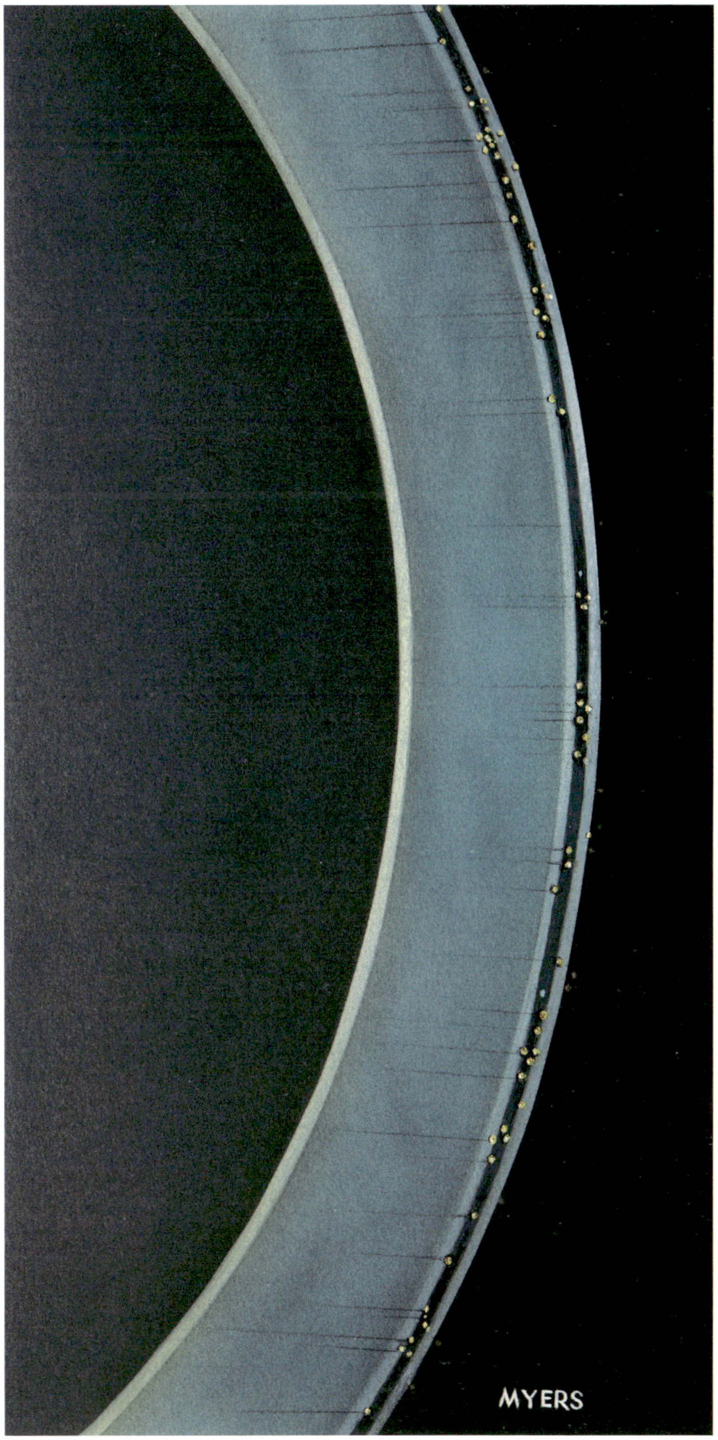
MYERS

PLATES 39 & 40

X-Linked Ichthyosis

These paintings demonstrate the filaform punctuate opacities in the deep stroma at the pre-Descemet membrane level, recognized in X-linked ichthyosis.

PLATE 39

This painting was reproduced in a black and white format as part of a report on the corneal changes of X-linked ichthyosis by Raymond Sever, MD (Chief Resident at the Bascom Palmer Eye Institute, 1966–67) and associates from the Department of Dermatology at the University of Miami School of Medicine in 1968. (Sever RJ, Frost P, Weinstein G. Eye changes in ichthyosis. JAMA 1968; 206:2283-2286). The deposits tend to be distributed diffusely over the whole posterior cornea, and in some were recognized in patches. The authors mention that in transillumination, the irregular opacities are similar to the changes of Cornea Farinata (Plates 33 and 34), but that all patients with X-linked ichthyosis had more prominent lesions and that they were large enough to be seen by direct illumination at the slit lamp. An example of the close working relationship between the referring faculty member and Mr. Myers is documented in a letter contained in the Bascom Palmer Eye Institute archives on Mr. Myers' stationary to Dr. Sever dated Dec. 26, 1966: *Here is the new wide slit view of the dystrophy associated with ichthyosis. For reasons of the loss of definition in the reproduction (photography and offset printing) I don't recommend making the precipitates any greyer than they are now for fear that they would not show at all. However, if after the slides and photos are made-you want them greyed down more- I will be glad to do it. Sincerely- Jack Myers.*

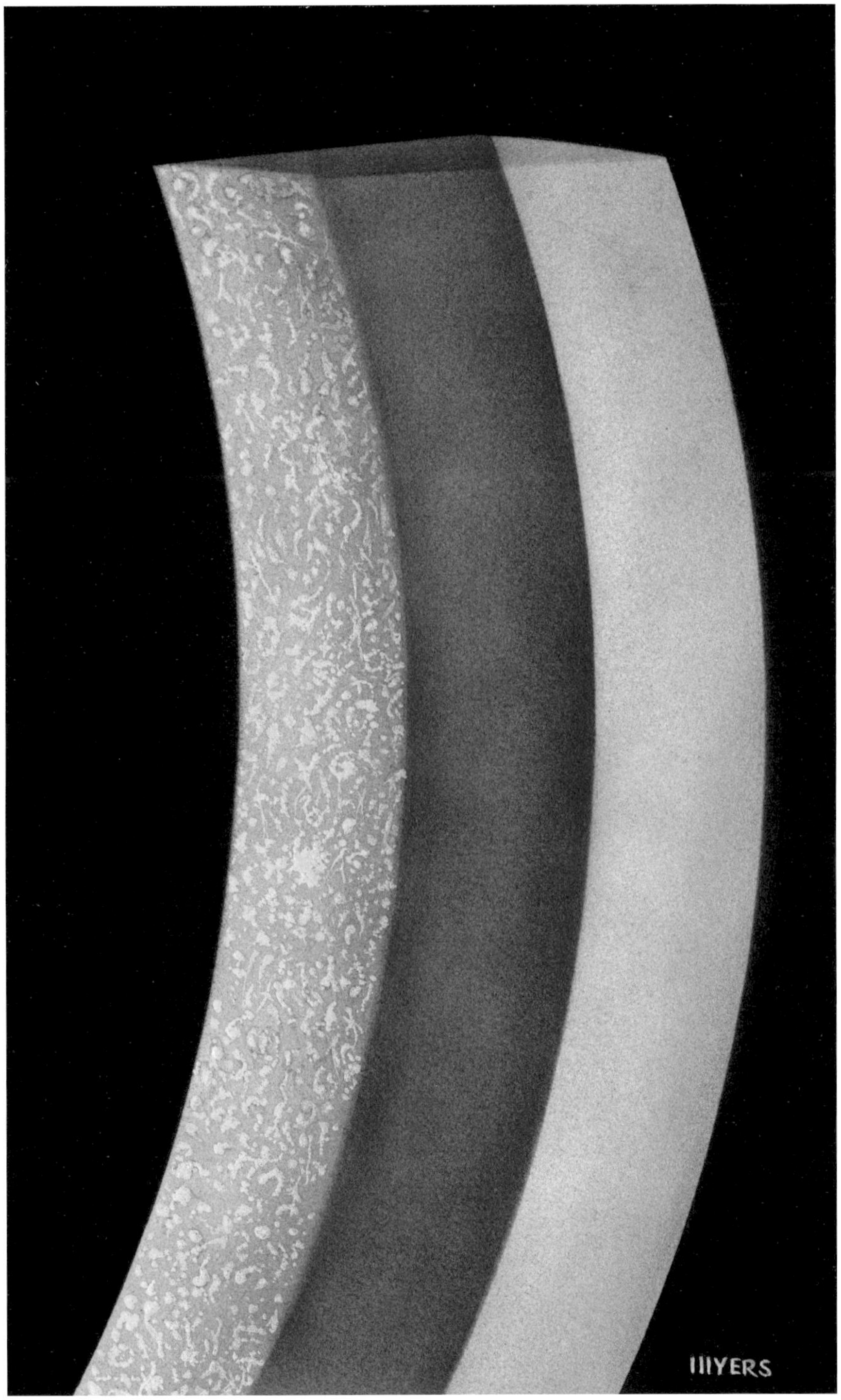
MYERS

PLATE 40

This illustration is from the reported series of patients but was not reproduced and probably represents a different patient from Plate 39. It clearly demonstrates the deep distribution of corneal opacities at the level of Descemet membrane. As mentioned in Severs et al.'s report, that area of the cornea is derived embryologically from mesoderm, in contrast to skin, which is of ectodermal origin. It was not known whether the opacities represent deposits of some substance or changes in the physical properties of corneal tissue.

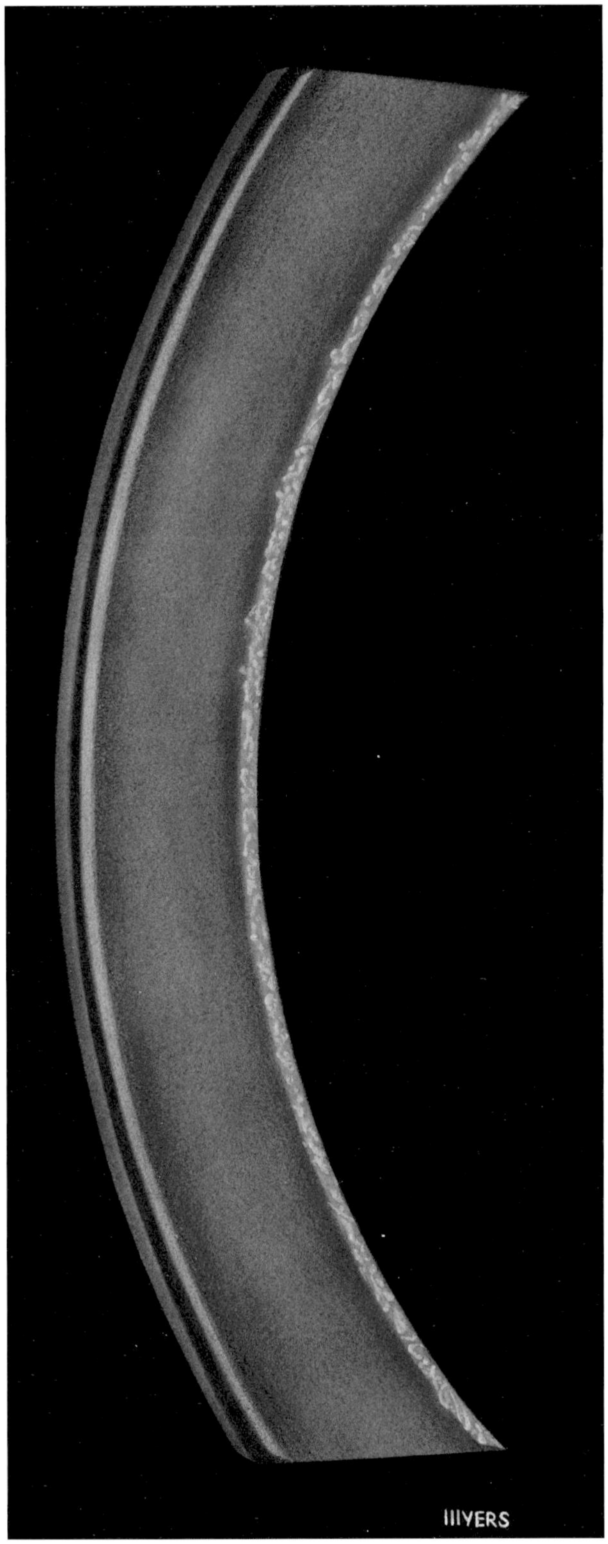
MYERS

PLATES 41 – 43

Chlorpromazine Deposition

Chronic use of the phenothiazine derivative, chlorpromazine, as a tranquilizing agent to treat schizophrenia may result in the deposition of amber-colored pigment on the posterior surface of the cornea and anterior lens capsule.

PLATE 41

Phenothiazine-related keratopathy is characterized by deposition of pigment on the corneal endothelial surface. Presumably, the chlorpromazine deposition is related to longstanding use of this phenothiazine derivative with substantial chronic circulating levels of the agent in the anterior chamber fluid. This painting demonstrates diffuse deposition localized to the posterior corneal surface.

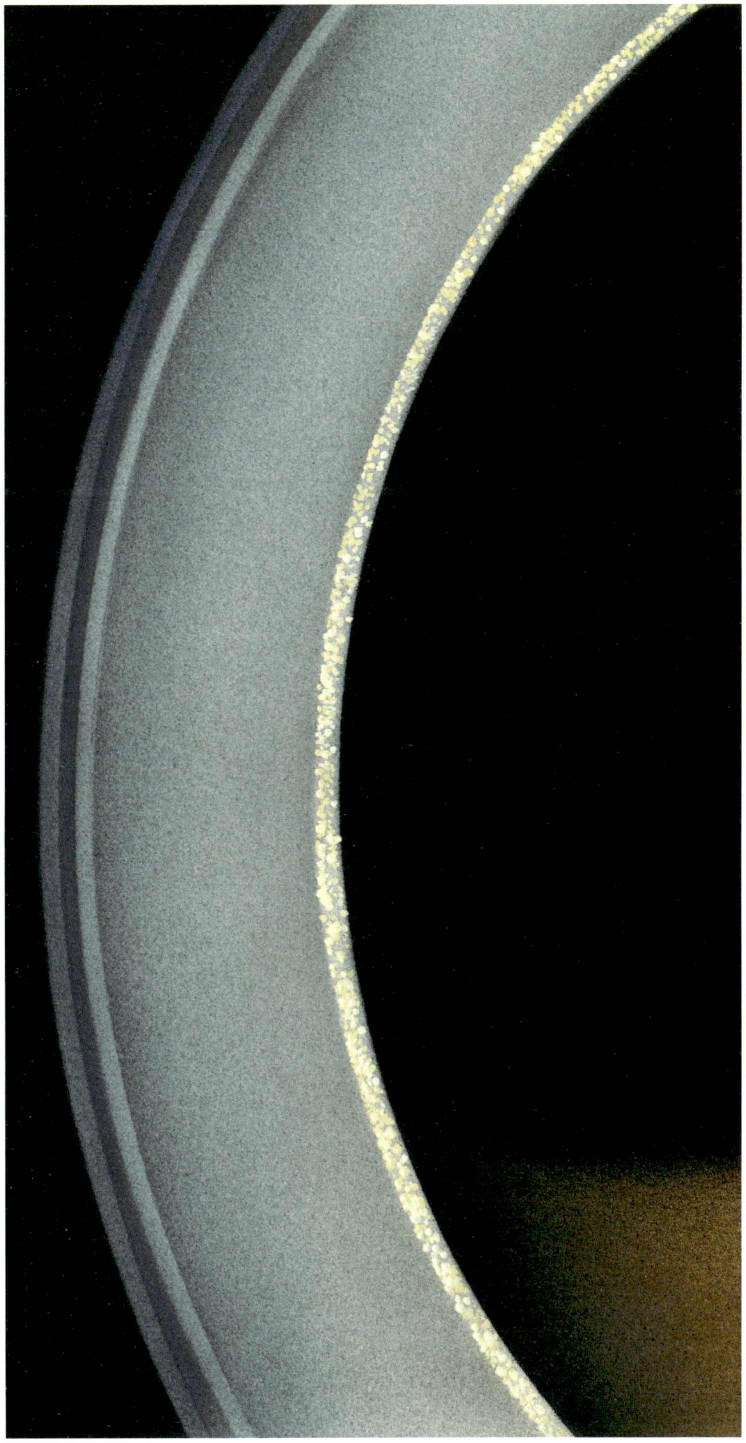

PLATE 42

Deposition of circulating chlorpromazine products result in the amber pigmentary changes on the anterior lens capsule. It is likely that the pigment is deposited on the surface, rather than incorporated into the capsule.

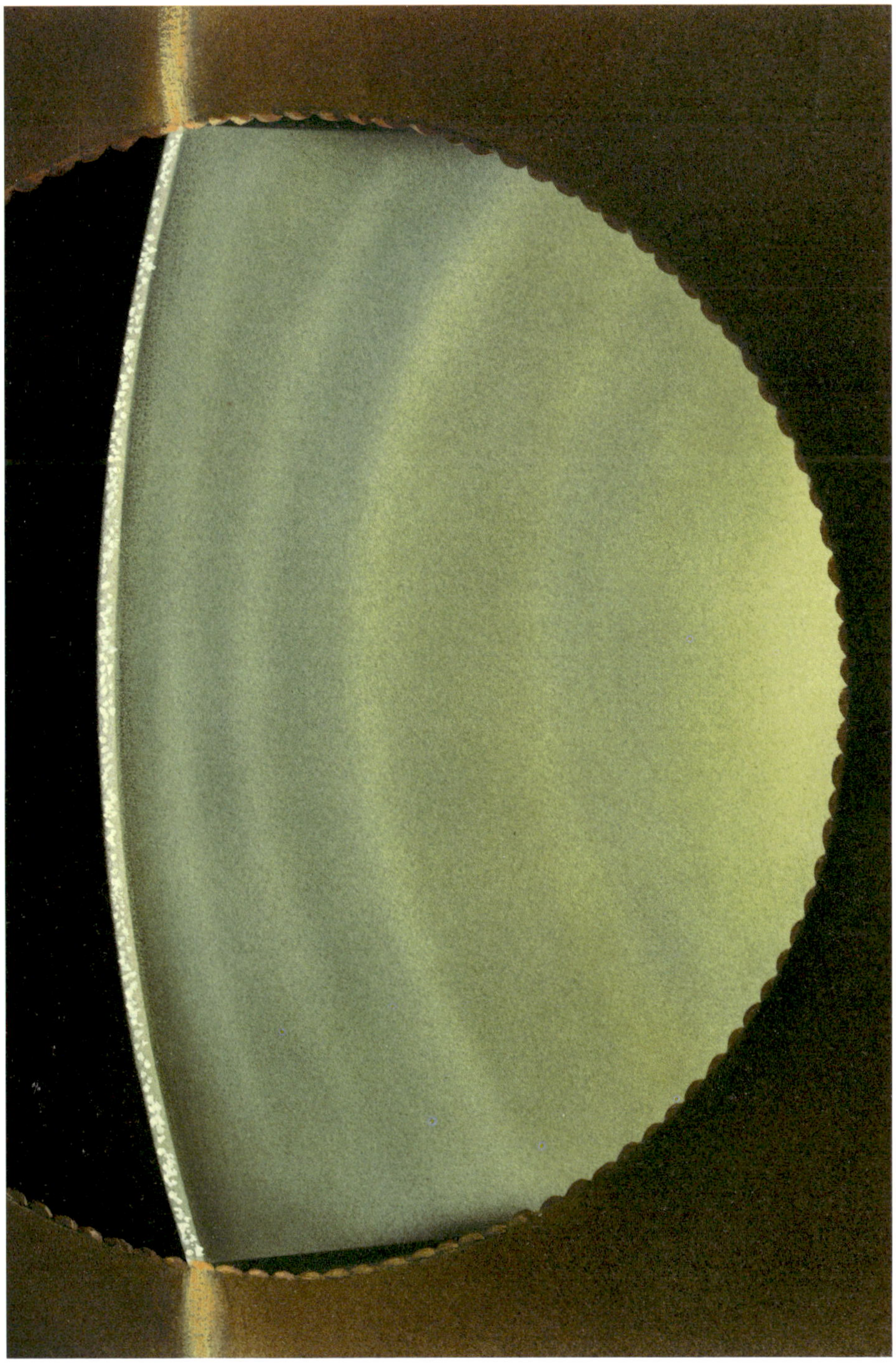

PLATE 43

This painting beautifully illustrates a stellate or floral pattern of pigment deposition on the anterior lens capsule.

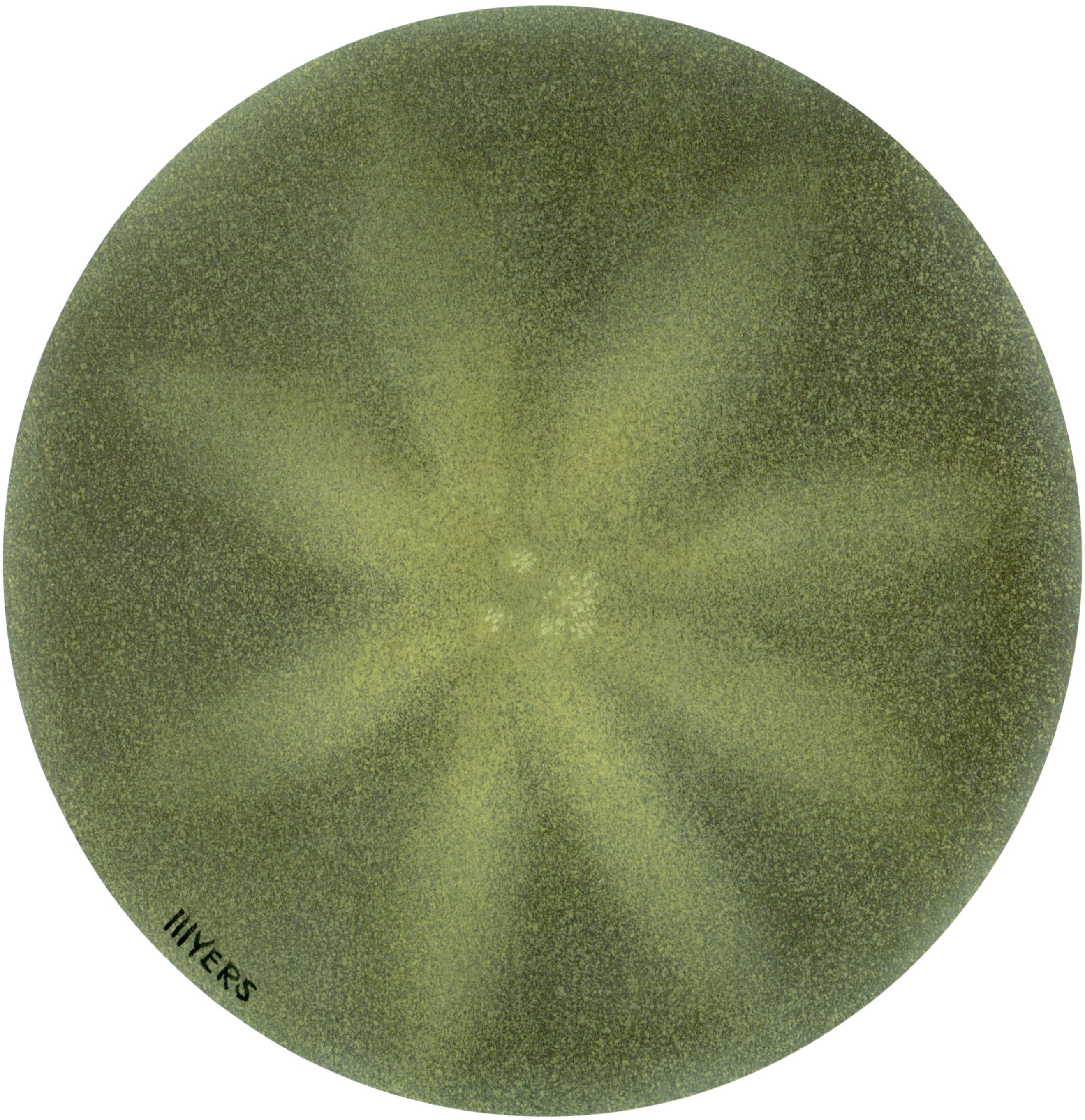
MYERS

PLATE 44

Cleft in Lens

This painting illustrates a most unusual crack or cleft in the middle of the lens nucleus separating the anterior and posterior halves, associated with a mild degree of cataract. Water clefts are not uncommon in the presence of cataracts, usually located in the lens cortex, but are most unusual in the adult nucleus. The clefts are thought to represent a disruption in the lens fiber layers and have been described following trauma. We only know that this patient was diabetic.

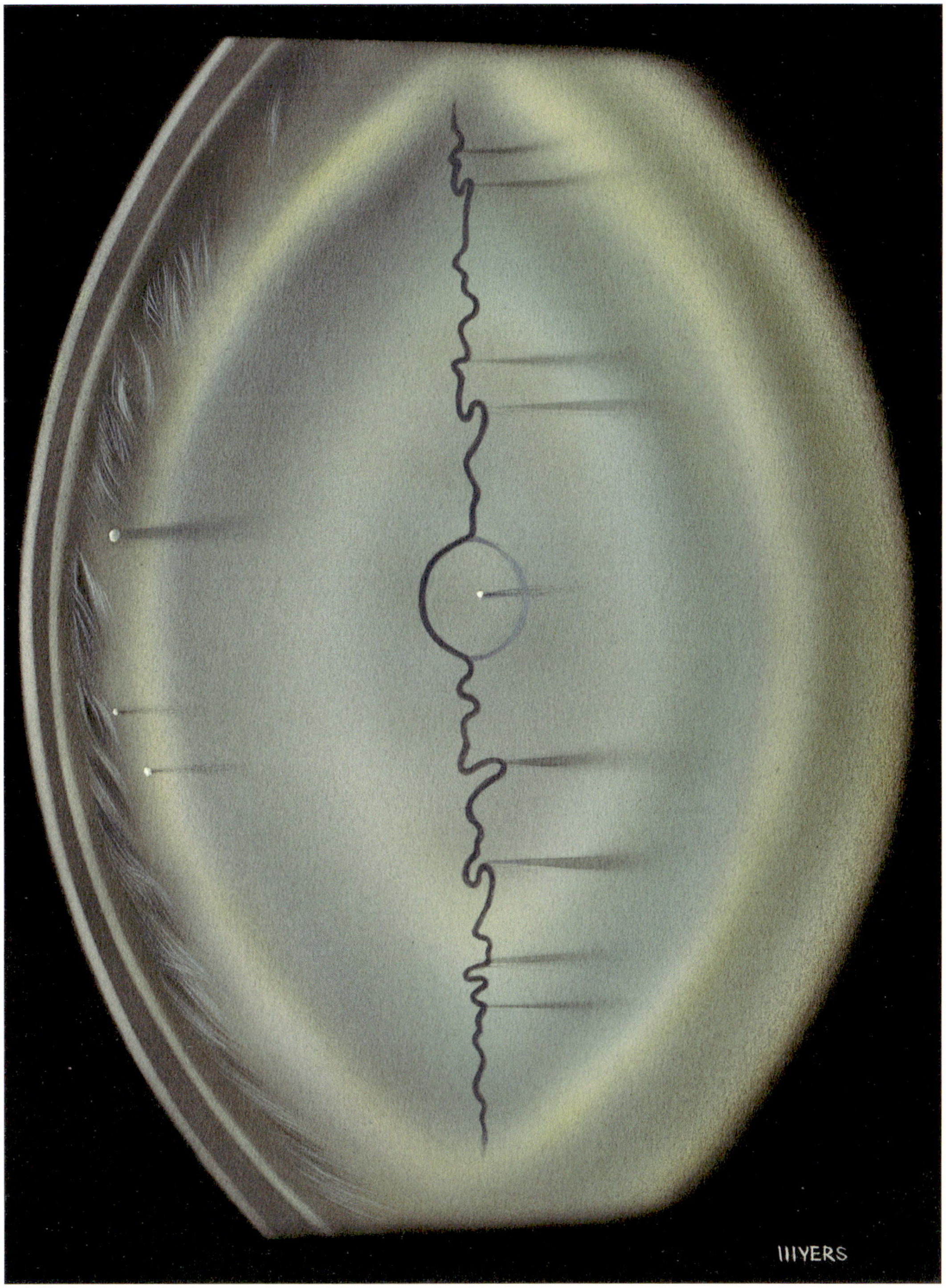
MYERS

PLATES 45 – 47

Posterior Lentiglobus

Posterior lentiglobus is a congenital lens anomaly characterized by a weakness or thinning of the posterior lens capsule, with ectasia and bowing of the posterior capsule and lens contents. In this bilateral and relatively symmetrical case, there is probably an acquired element that has led to further opacity of the lens substance.

PLATE 45

This illustration of the right eye demonstrates an intact anterior capsular slit-beam view with prominent posterior herniation of the lens capsule. Most of the lens opacity or cataract involves the posterior ecstatic portion of the lens, contiguous with the capsular weakness.

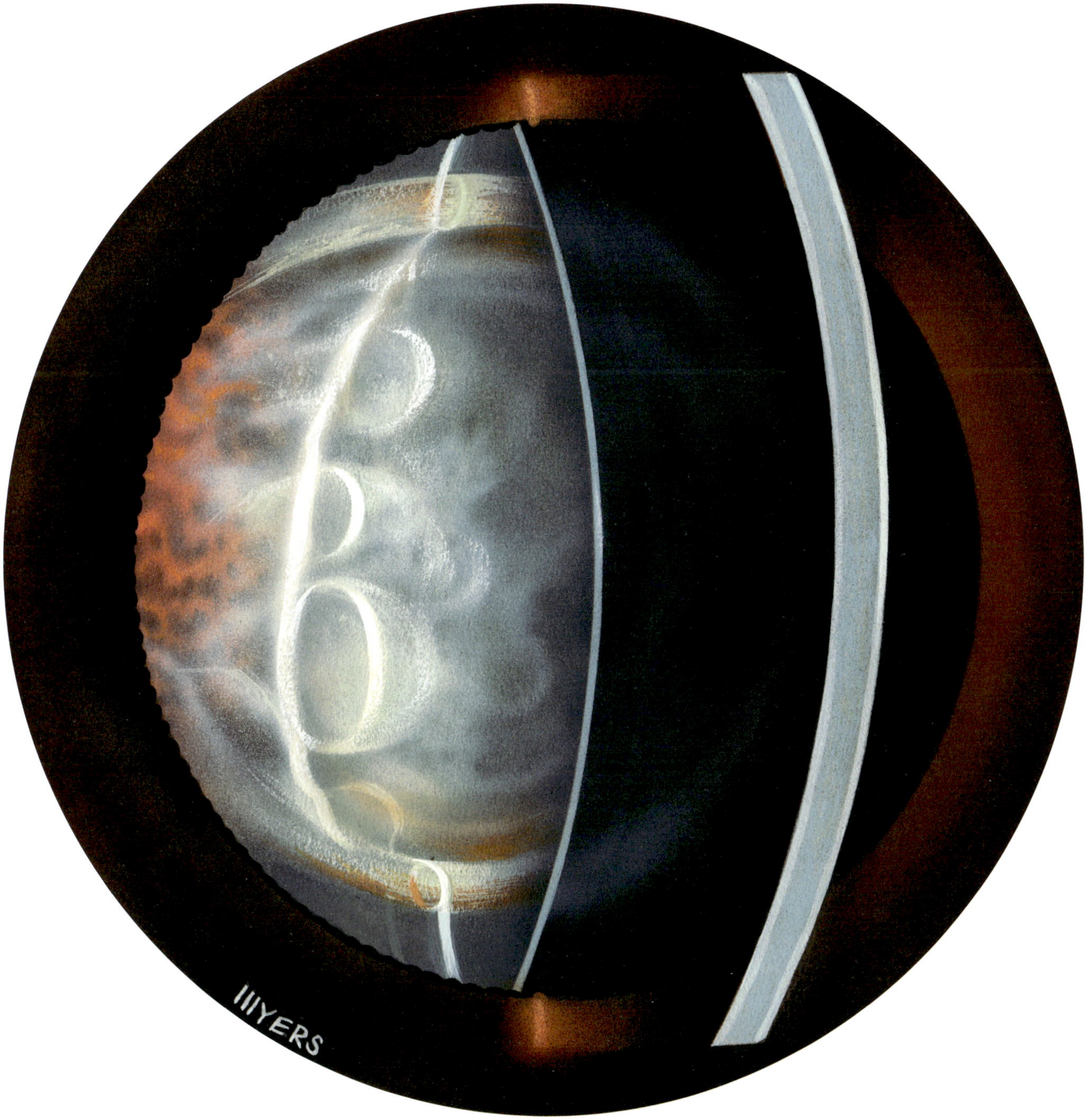

PLATE 46

The painting of the left eye shows a similar intact anterior capsule, but with even more prominent ectasia of the posterior capsule. However, the lens opacity does not extend to the periphery in either eye and allows for visualization of the red reflex with transillumination.

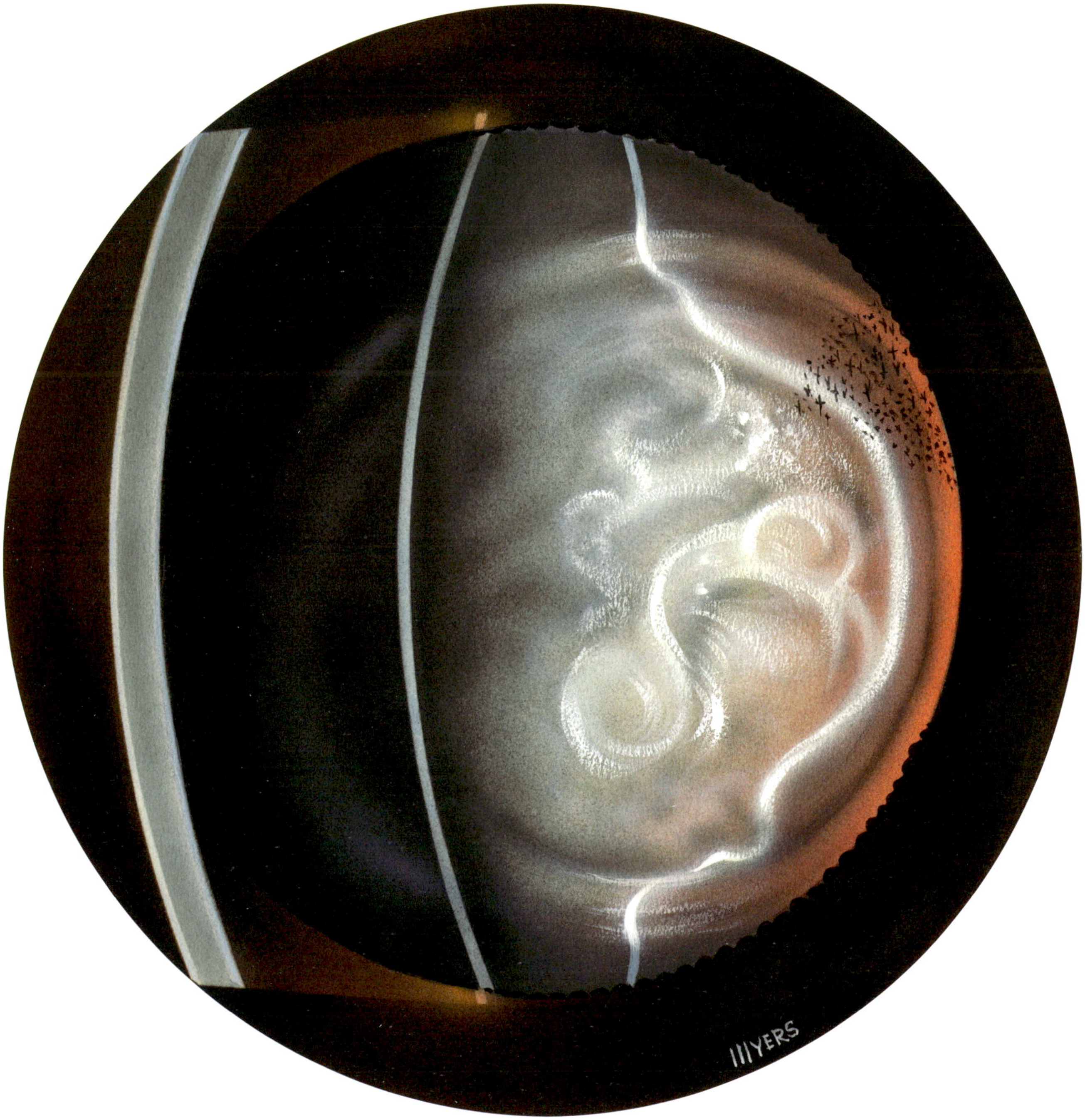
MYERS

PLATE 47

This retroillumination view of the left eye beautifully captures the intriguing swirl-like pattern of the lentiglobus and cataract against the red fundus reflex.

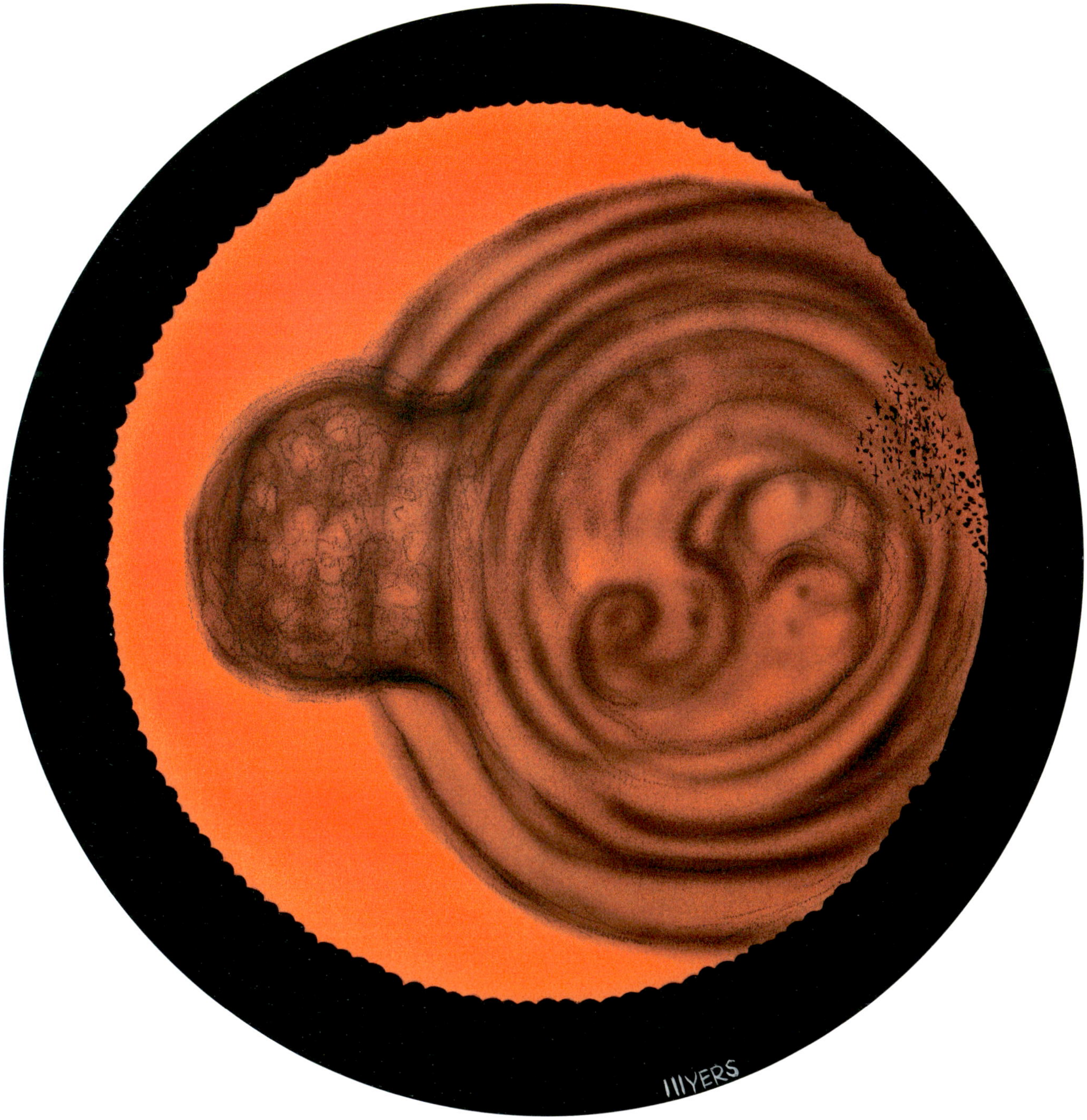
MYERS

PLATES 48 – 50

Christmas Tree Cataract

PLATE 48

A stellate pattern of polychromatic opacities in the anterior lens cortex suggests holiday ornaments. Typically, the predominant colors are characterized by gold linear crystals, with the "colored lights" in cerulean and shades of red. The stellate appearance is unusual, but probably represents cortical lens clefts and opacities as part of the cataract.

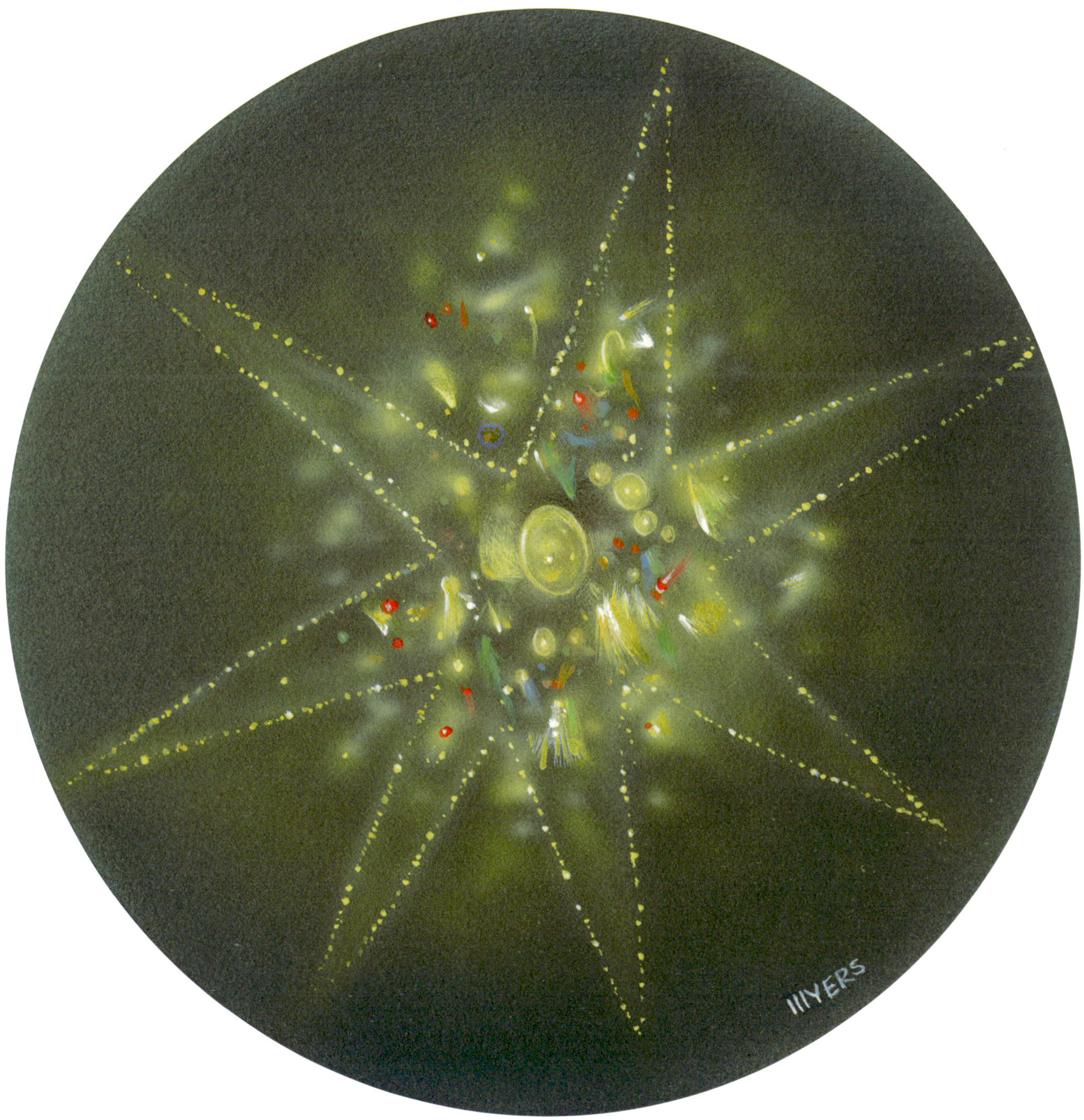
MYERS

PLATE 49

The slit-beam view localizes the polychromatic lens opacities to the posterior cortex in the axial or central portions of the lens. Mr. Myers was able to capture specific opacities which one can identify in carefully comparing plates 48 and 49.

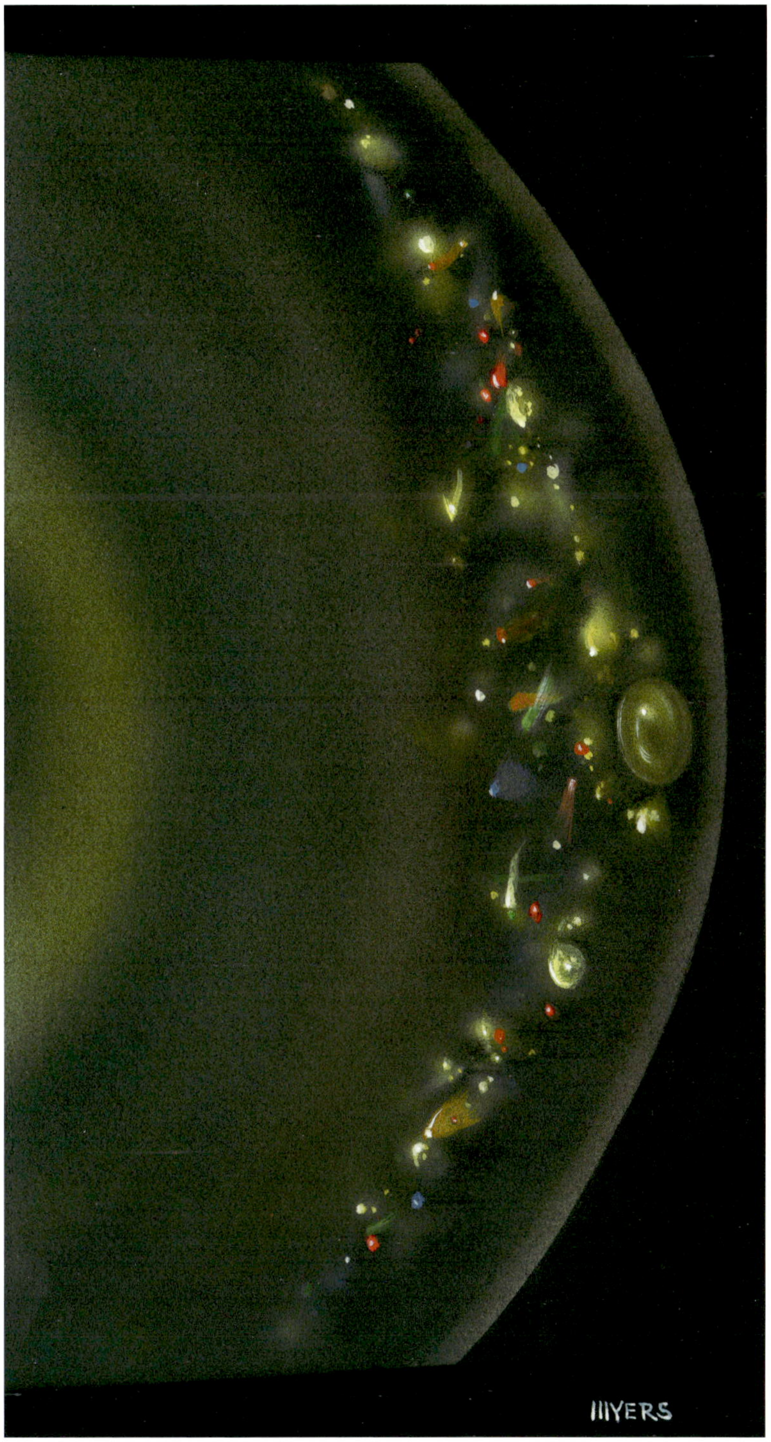
MYERS

PLATE 50

This slit-beam view is from the same left eye, but appears to illustrate the anterior cortical portions of the lens with the lens epithelium under or inside the capsule. The colorful opacities are much less prominent in the anterior lens than in the posterior cortex, as demonstrated in Plate 49.

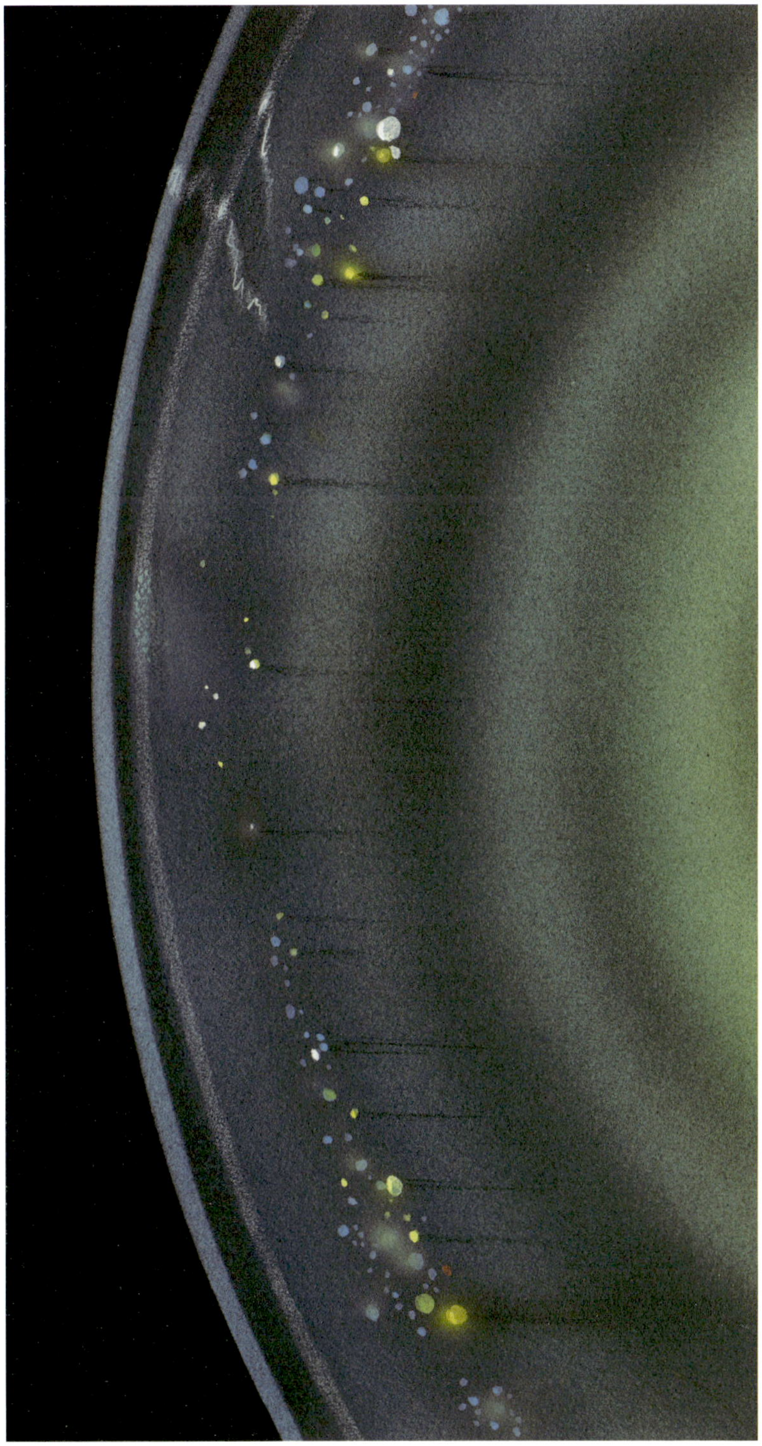

PLATES 51–58

Primary Amyloidosis of the Vitreous and Surgical Treatment

These paintings illustrate the vitreous changes associated with the rarely recognized diagnosis of primary amyloidosis of the eye. The changes are characterized by the progressive development of gray-white opacities which involve the entire vitreous framework and became so dense that the vision in these two cases was reduced to counting fingers, hand movements, and only light perception in one eye. The opacities may prevent visualization of the retina and are characteristic in their bilateral appearance. The fibrilla of the vitreous gel become thickened and opaque, with tiny round opacities attached to the fibrils.

These paintings were crafted to illustrate a new surgical treatment for amyloidosis of the vitreous which was reported by Kasner and associates from the Bascom Palmer Eye Institute at the annual meeting of the American Academy of Ophthalmology and Otolaryngology in Chicago, Illinois, USA in 1967, and published in 1968 (Kasner D, Miller GR, Taylor WH, Sever RJ, Norton EWD. Surgical Treatment of Amyloidosis of the Vitreous. Trans Am Acad Ophthalmol Otolaryngol 1968; 72:410-418).

PLATE 51

Case 1, right eye. The patient was a 67 year old with a ten-year history of progressive visual loss in both eyes. Vision was hand movements. The vitreous was described as veil-like and opaque with gray strands filling the vitreous cavity, uniform in density and moveable; the opacities precluded a view of the retina.

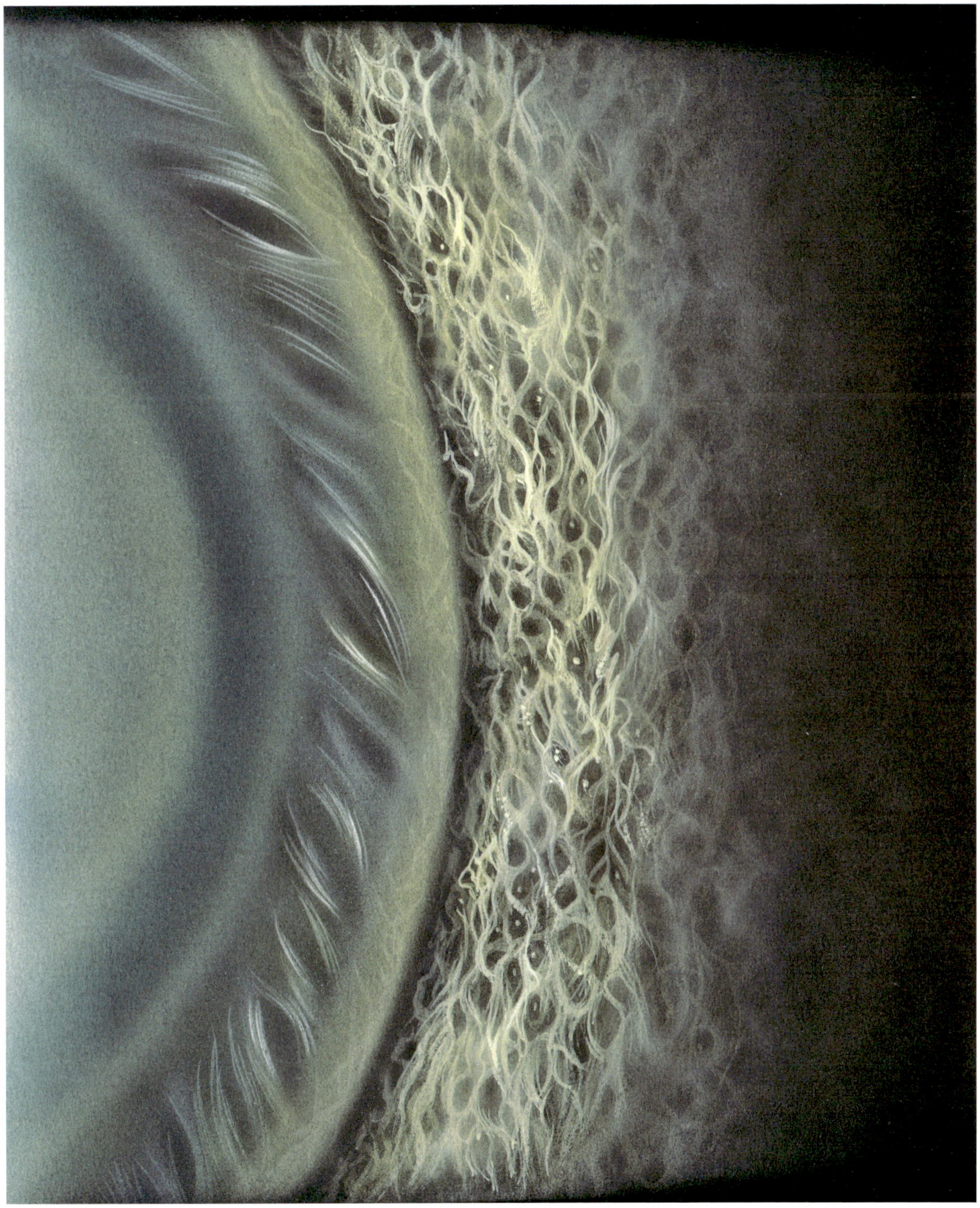

PLATE 52

Case 1, left eye. Vision in this eye was counting fingers at three feet and only the disc outline could be seen due to the vitreous opacities. The description of the vitreous was similar to that in Plate 51.

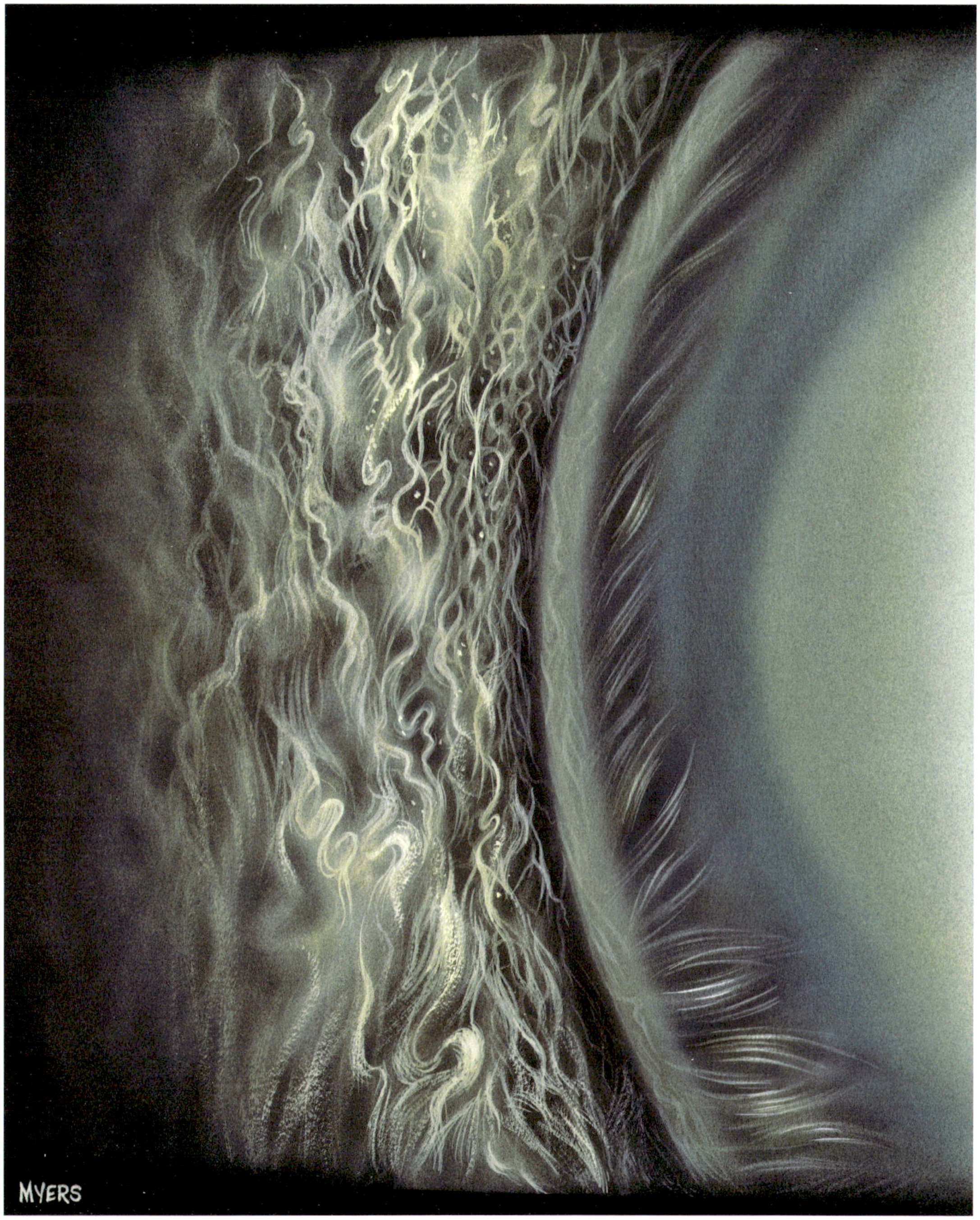
MYERS

PLATE 53

This painting is from Case 1, but was not included in the publication. The vitreous opacities in the slit-beam view directly behind the lens appear to be even more dense than in Plates 51 and 52.

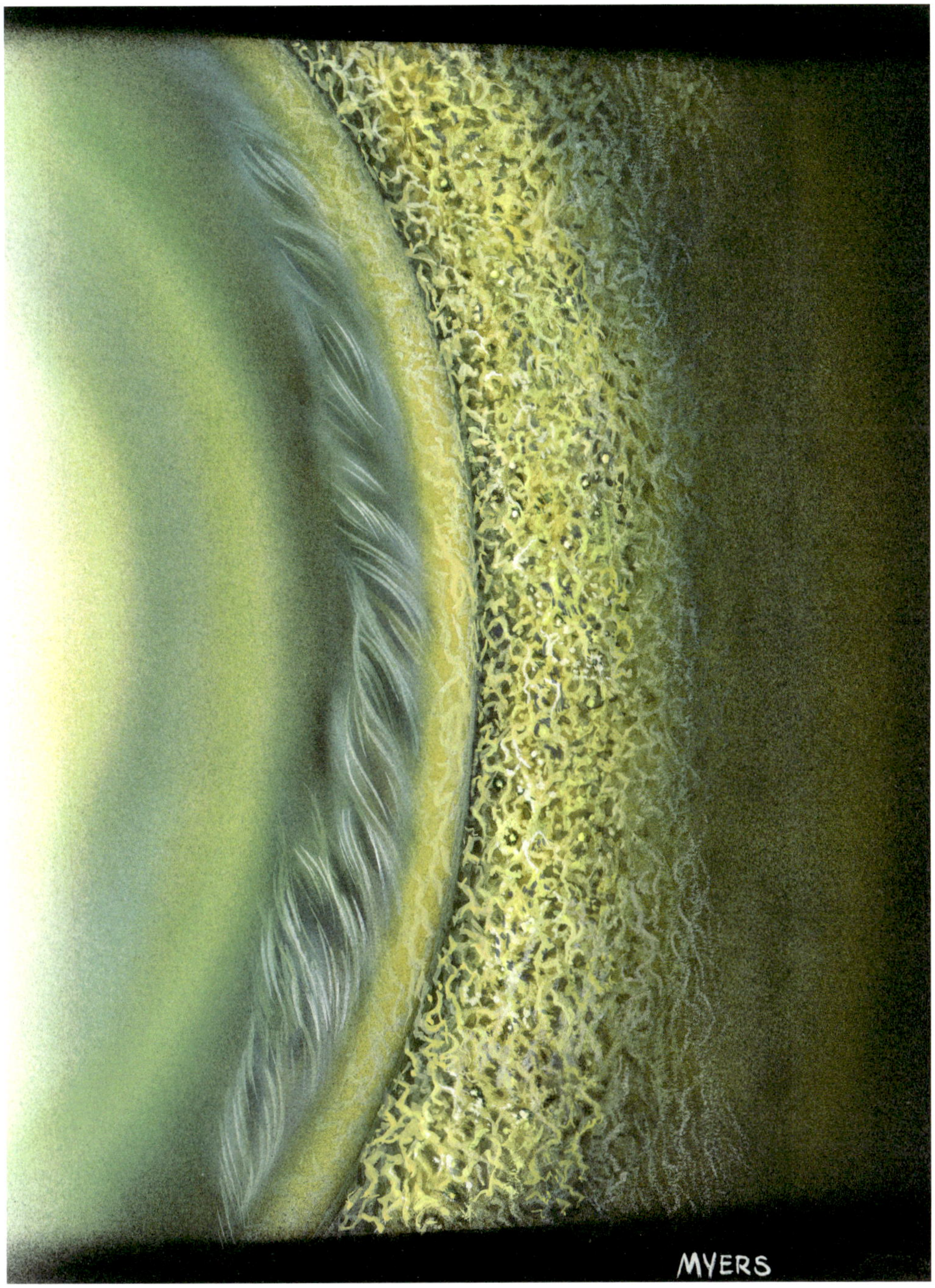
MYERS

PLATE 54

This is a diagrammatic illustration of the surgical approach and technique of excising the vitreous in the right eye of Case 1.

54a. An "open-sky" approach was used in which a 300-degree corneal incision was made, the cornea was then folded back, an iridectomy performed, and the lens removed intracapsularly.

54b. The vitreous was excised by grasping formed vitreous with a smooth forceps and cutting with scissors. Fluid vitreous was absorbed with cellulose sponges. The excision continued posteriorly until the macula and optic disc were uncovered. Kasner et al. stated: "The procedure produced a tunnel approximately 1 cm in diameter through the opaque vitreous to the posterior pole." The corneal wound was then sutured in place. After eight months, the vision was corrected to 20/70 at distance and 20/30 at near.

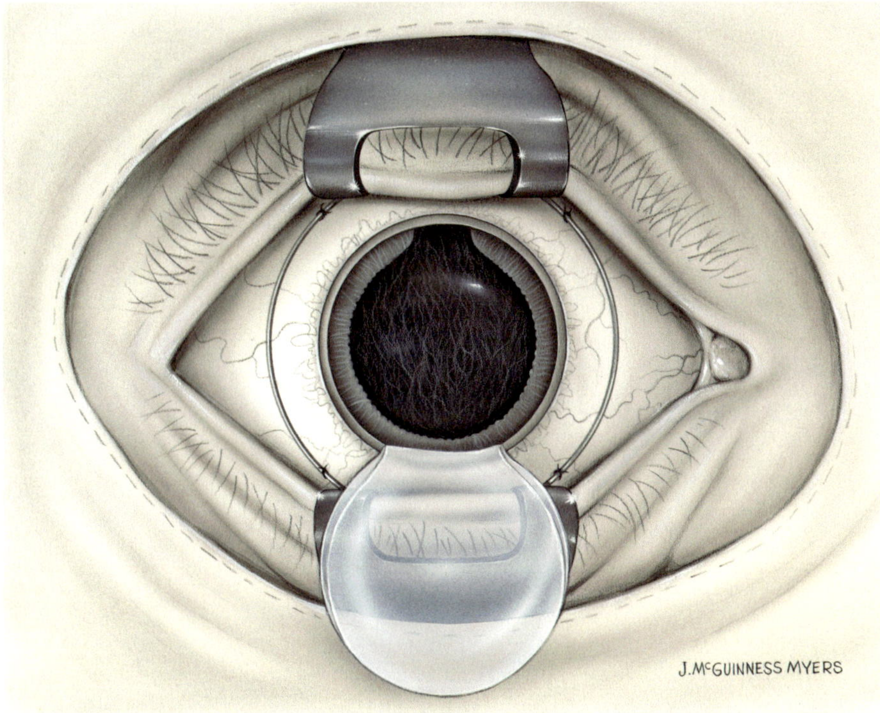

54a

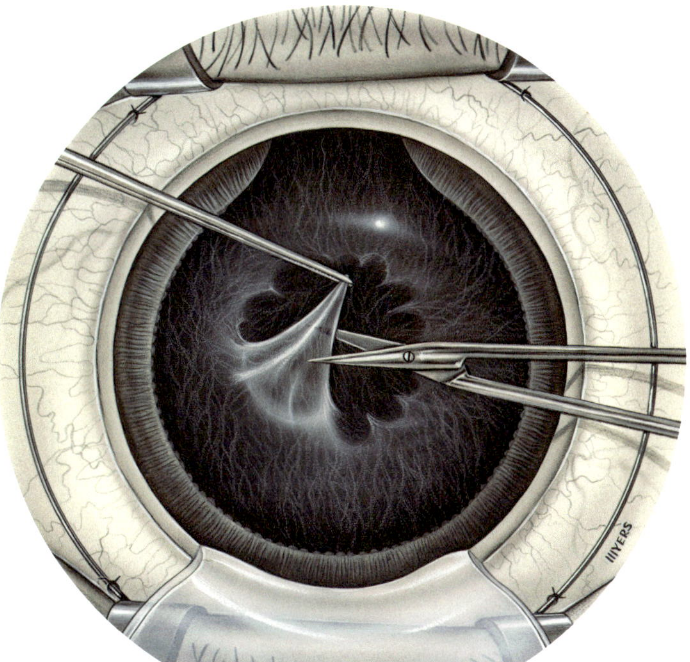

54b

PLATE 55

This painting demonstrates the postoperative view of the retina with the silhouette of the residual vitreous after the core vitrectomy was completed.

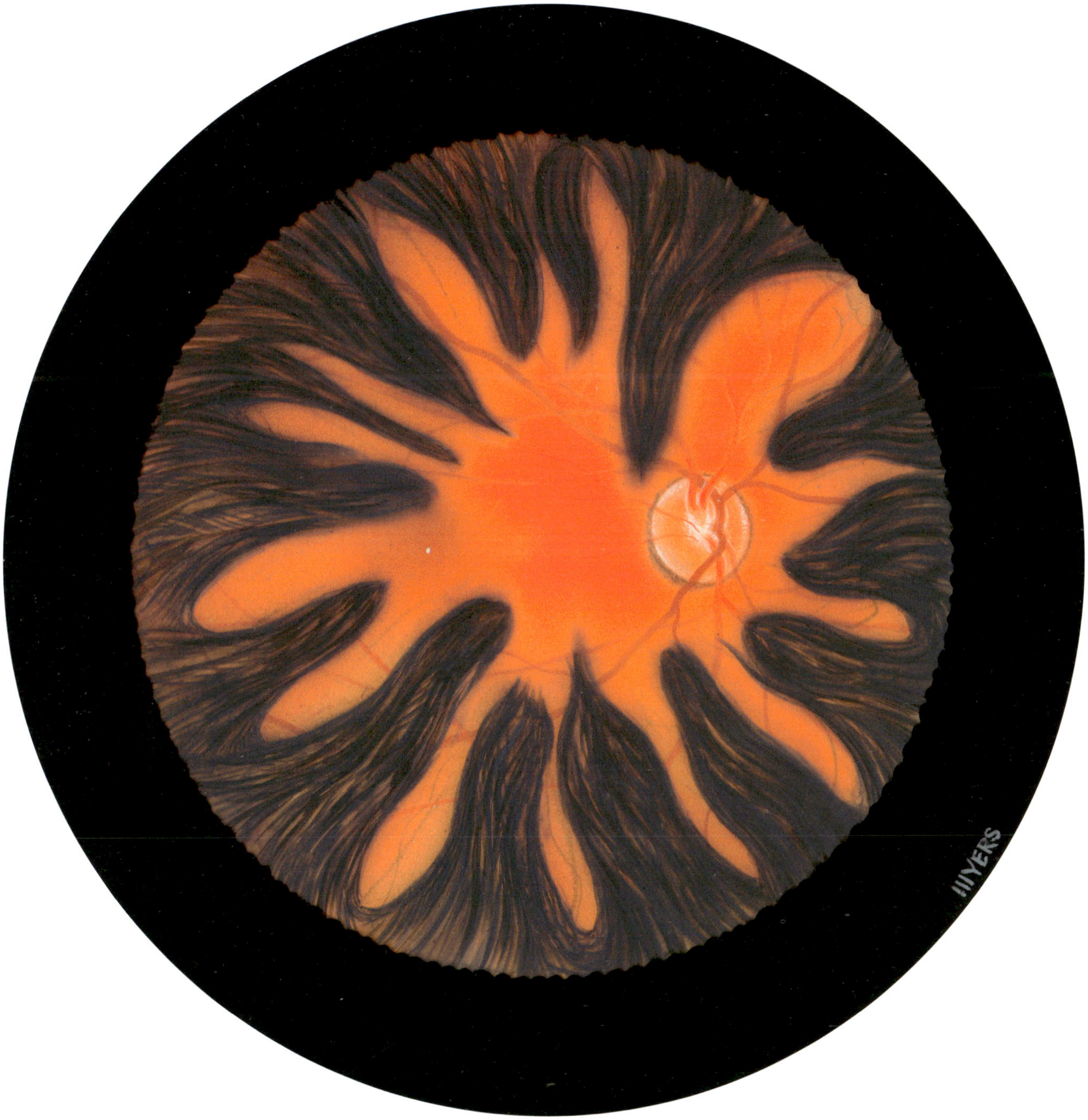
MYERS

PLATE 56

Case 2, right eye. This patient was a 62 year old with a 4 to 5 year progressive visual loss in both eyes with vision of counting fingers at one foot. A systemic diagnosis of primary amyloidosis was made and as in Case 1, showed amyloidosis from the excised vitreous.

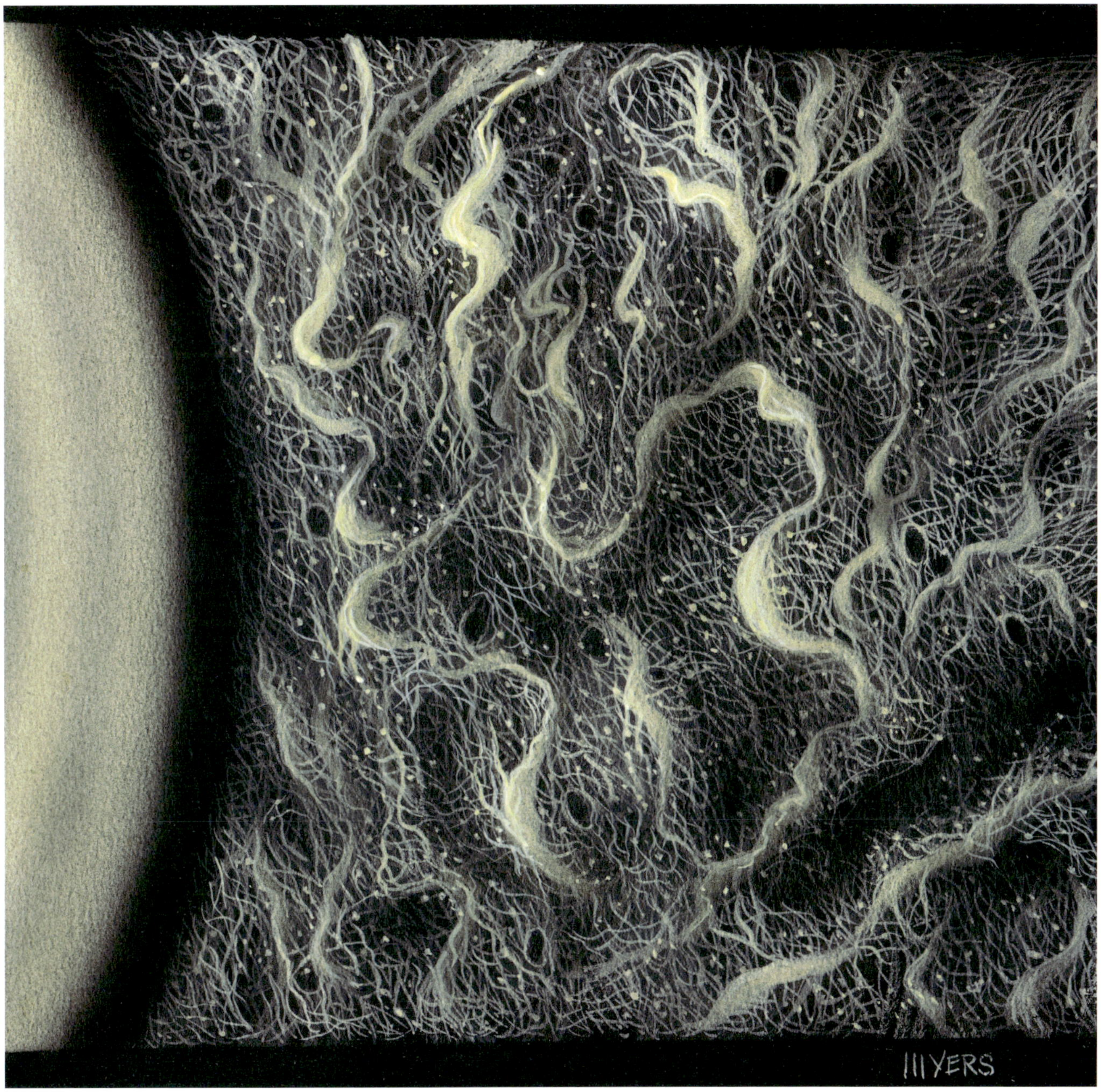
MYERS

PLATE 57

Case 2, left eye. The vitreous opacities were nearly identical in both eyes and similar to Case 1. The patient underwent vitrectomy by the same approach as in Case 1. Two months following surgery, the vision was corrected to 20/40 with a contact lens.

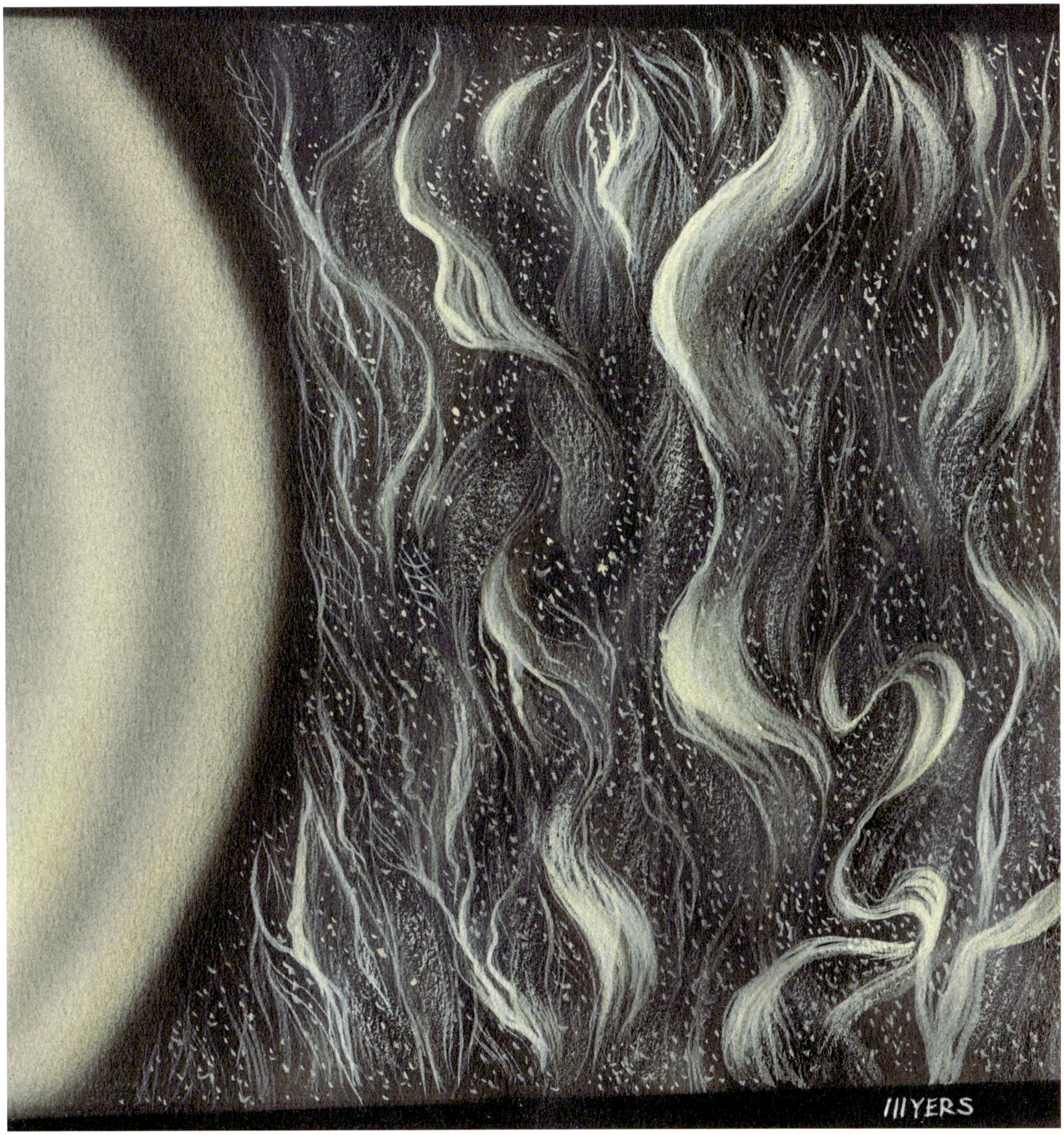
MYERS

PLATE 58

This painting of Case 2 was not included in the publication, but clearly demonstrates the classic vitreous opacities of primary amyloidosis.

The surgical approach to vitrectomy was revolutionized in the spring of 1970, when Robert Machemer, MD performed the world's first pars plana vitrectomy with a mechanical vitrector referred to as the VISC (Vitreous Infusion Suction Cutter), which he developed in collaboration with the biomedical engineer, Jean-Marie Parel, PhD at the Bascom Palmer Eye Institute.

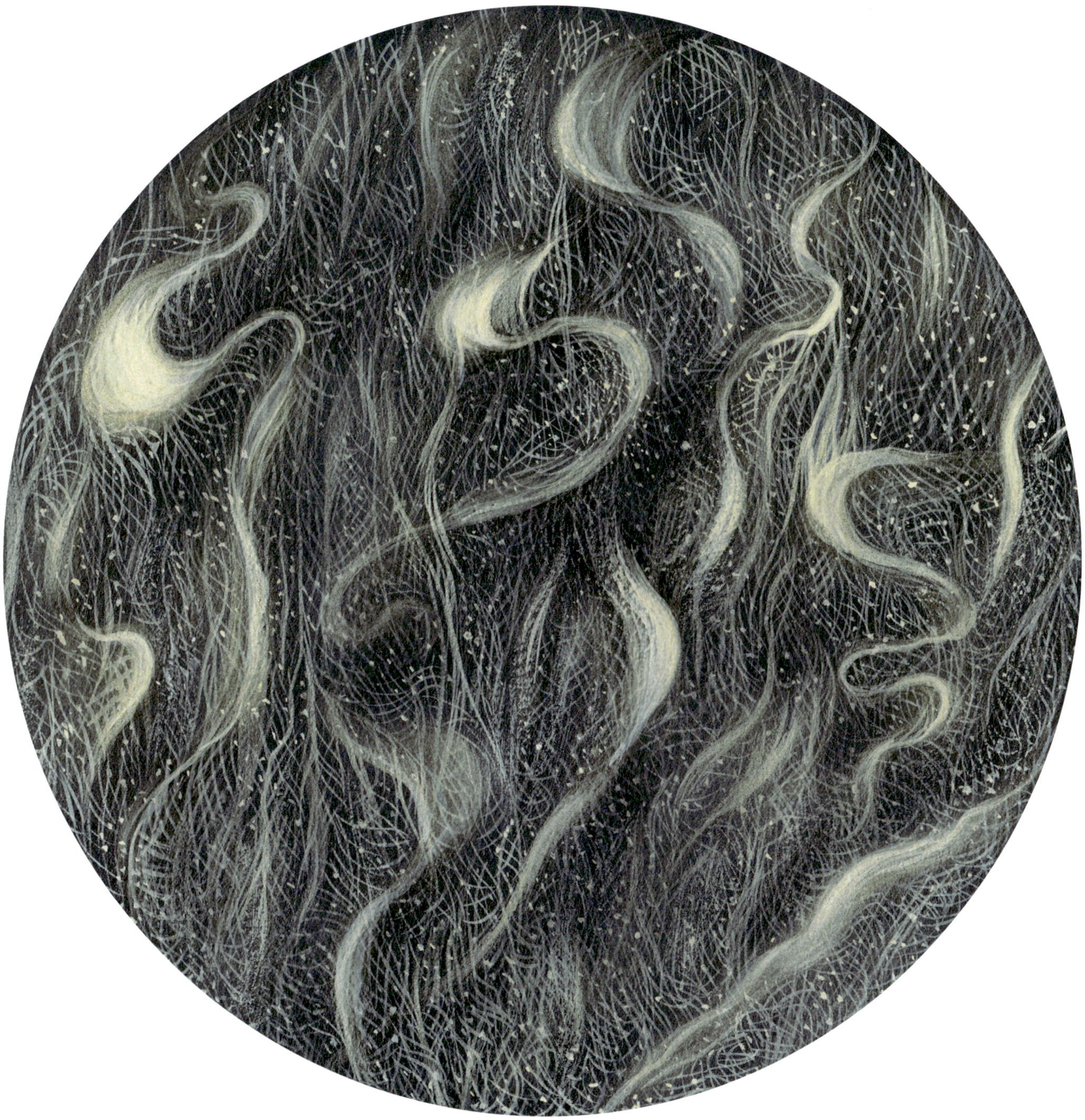

PLATES 59 – 61

Cystoid Macular Edema

These three paintings, done on paper on board, are the only ones that Mr. Myers completed at BPEI that have been published in color. They appear in the classic article by Gass and Norton describing the fluorescein fundoscopic and angiographic features of cystoid macular edema following cataract surgery (Gass JDM, Norton EWD. Cystoid macular edema and papilledema following cataract extraction. Arch Ophthalmol 1966; 76:646-661).

PLATE 59

The ophthalmoscopic appearance of cystoid macular edema following cataract surgery, reproduced from the original photograph of this specific patient.

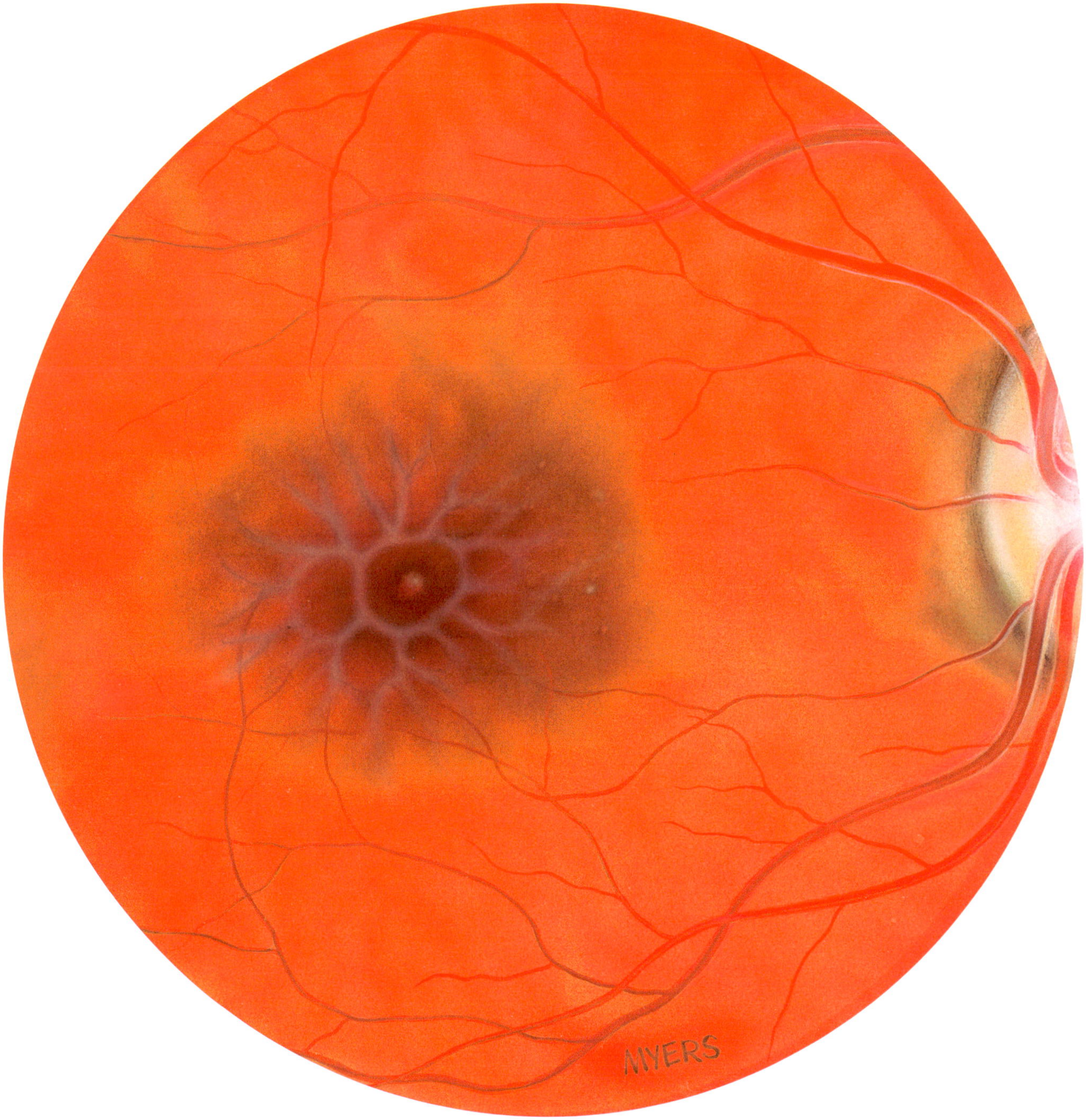
MYERS

PLATE 60

The biomicroscopic appearance of cystoid macular edema demonstrating the elevated thickening and collection of fluid in the macula. This illustration was reproduced in black and white in Dr. Gass' classic atlas (Gass JDM. Stereoscopic Atlas of Macular Disease; a Funduscopic and Angiographic Presentation, 1st ed. St. Louis, CV Mosby, 1970).

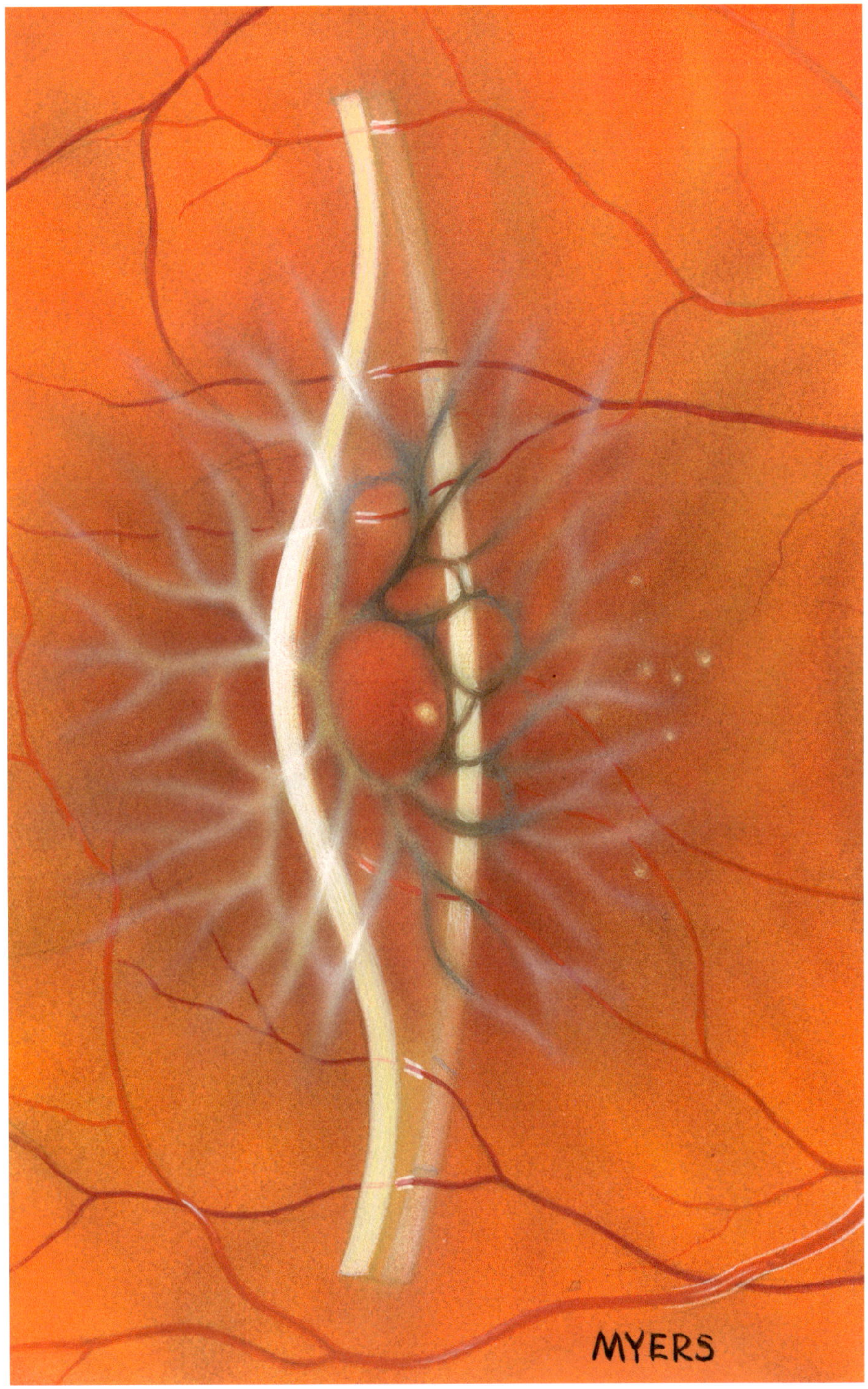
MYERS

PLATE 61

The fluorescein angiographic appearance of cystoid macular edema that is diagnostic of this condition. The specific recirculation phase fluorescein angiogram image that Myers based his painting on was photographed by Johnny Justice, Jr., a medical photographer who joined the Bascom Palmer Eye Institute in 1962 and who showed these photographs to Dr. Gass shortly after Dr. Gass joined the BPEI faculty in 1963. Mr. Justice worked closely with Dr. Gass pioneering the technique of fluorescein angiography, which allows vessels of the eye to be photographed in dynamic detail.

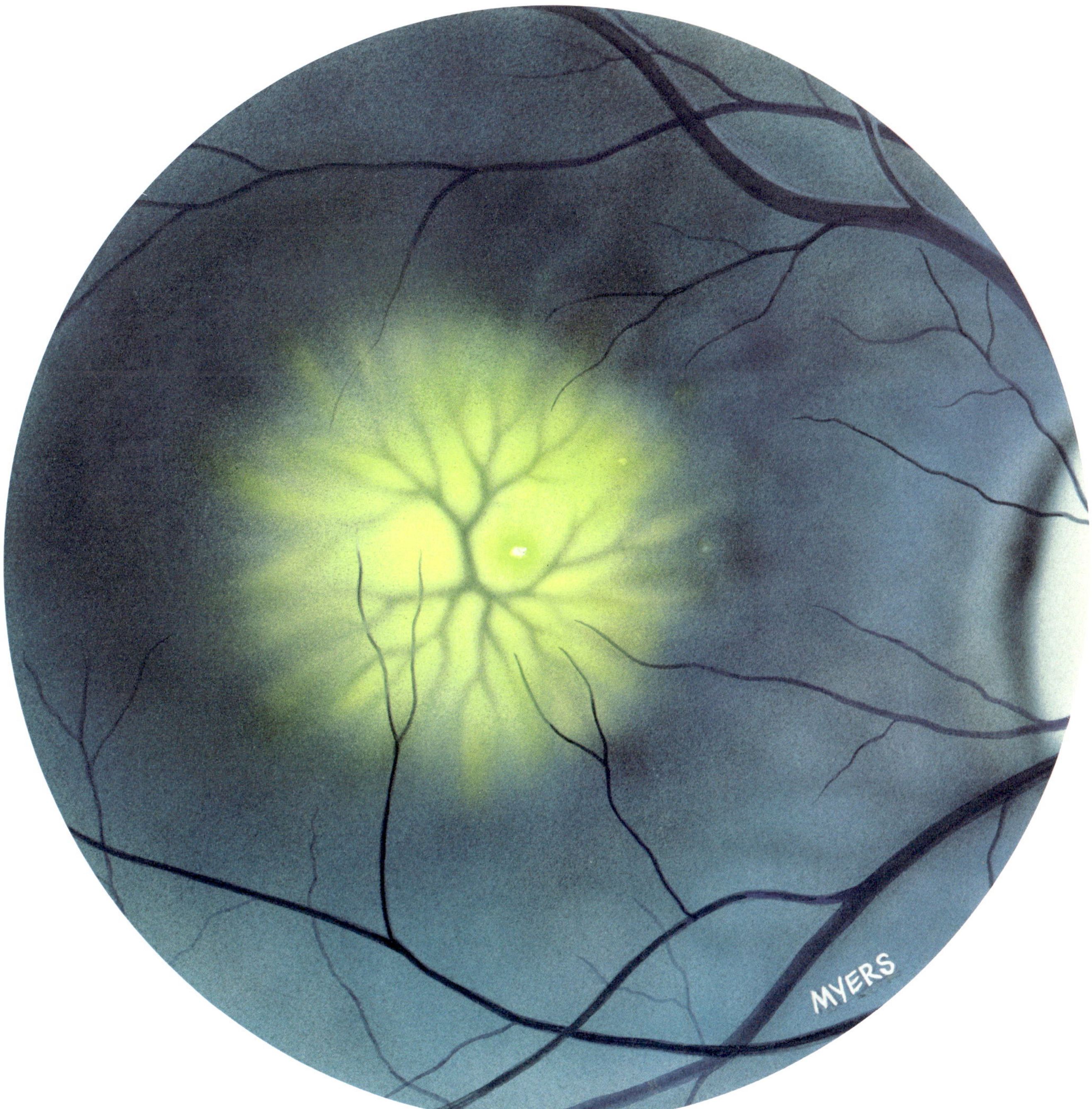
MYERS

PLATE 62

Epiretinal Membrane

These paintings demonstrate the appearance of an epiretinal membrane, which is also referred to more colloquially as a macular pucker. In addition to the deposition of contractile tissue on the surface of the retina, the retinal surface can become corrugated and irregular resulting in distorted vision.

62a. This painting represents the ophthalmoscopic appearance of an epiretinal membrane. Note the glistening tissue on the surface of the retina.

62b. In this painting, a partial posterior vitreous separation in the macular region is depicted along with a central opening in the posterior hyaloid. It is felt that a chronically adherent hyaloid attachment in the macula may be partly responsible for the development of an epiretinal membrane, which is subtly evident on the retinal surface. A normal macular contour is demonstrated with a preserved foveal depression centrally and a healthy-appearing retinal pigment epithelium and choriocapillaris being observed in the cross-section highlight. This patient is likely asymptomatic.

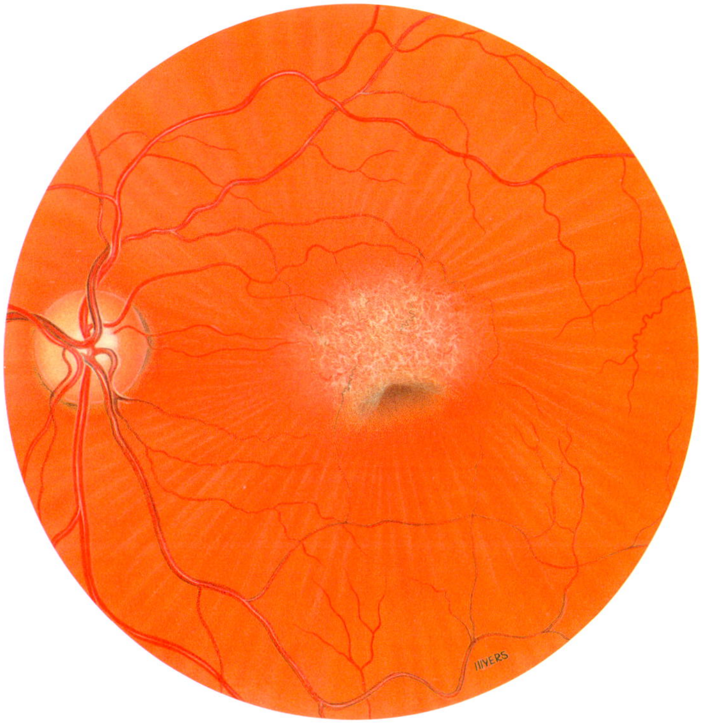

62a

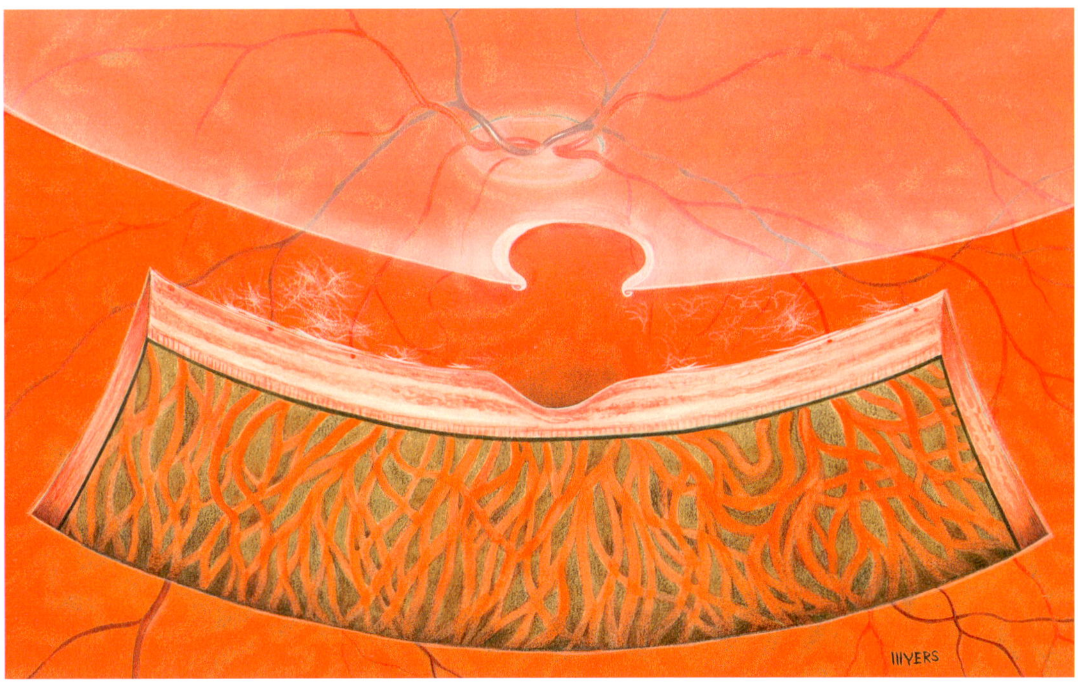

62b

PLATE 63

Epiretinal Membrane

In these paintings, Mr. Myers demonstrates a more significant ophthalmoscopic appearance of an epiretinal membrane. There is an increased level of macular distortion and vessel dystopia; therefore, these patients are more likely to be symptomatic.

63a. This painting depicts a diffuse epiretinal membrane affecting the temporal macular region with superficial fibrous tissue being seen extending vertically and obliquely and dragging the retinal vessels.

63b. Although glistening superficial fibrous tissue representing an epiretinal membrane is observed in the region abutting the fovea superiorly, the cross-sectional cutout image demonstrates a normal macular contour without retinal edema or loss of the foveal depression.

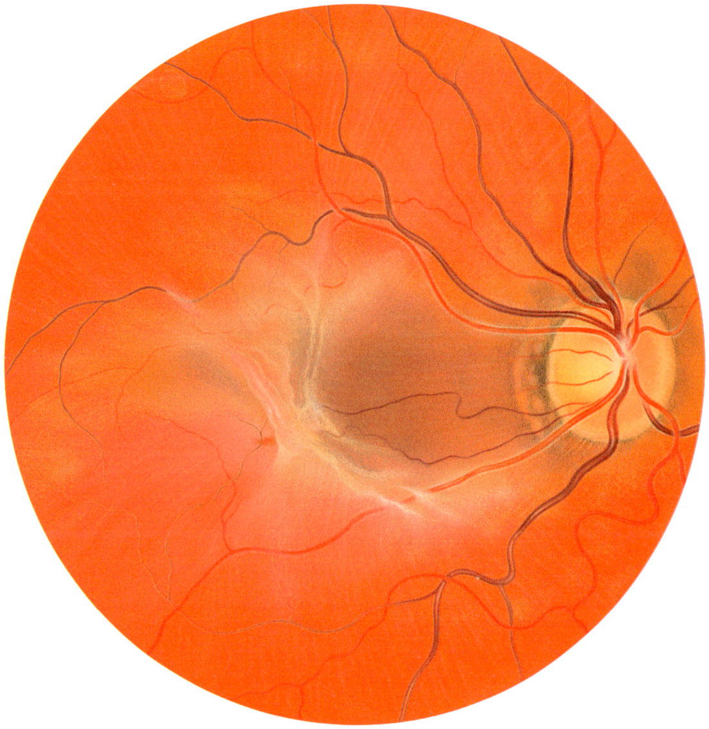

63a

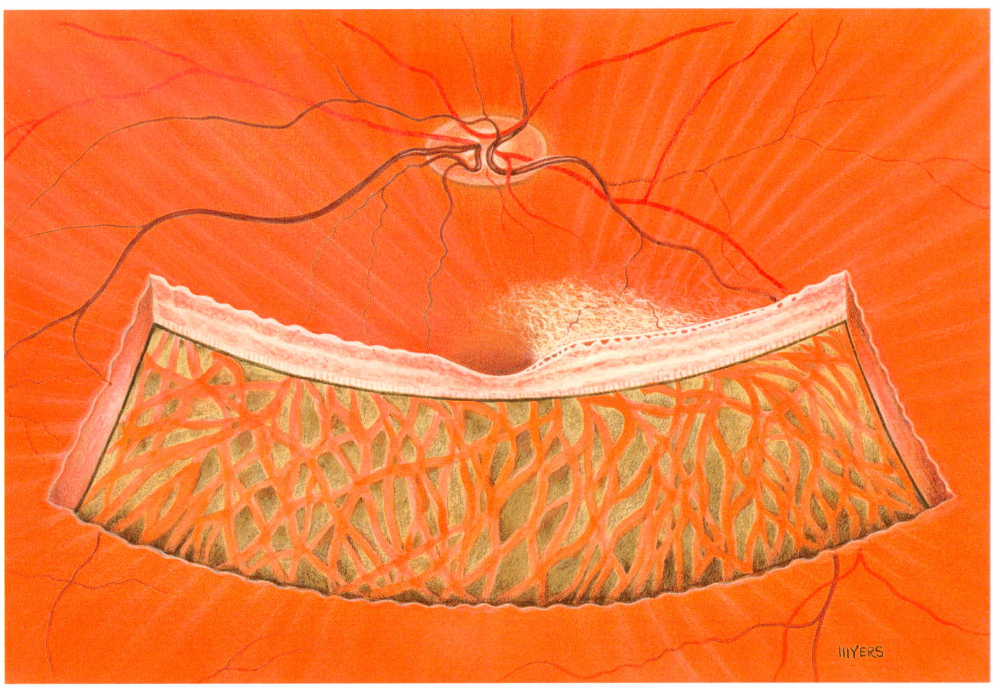

63b

PLATE 64

Combined Hamartoma of the Retina and Retinal Pigment Epithelium

A combined hamartoma of the retina and retinal pigment epithelium is demonstrated in these two paintings representing different vantage points in the same patient. This is a rare condition, thought to be congenital, in which tissue that normally resides in the retina and retinal pigment epithelium grows in an abnormal fashion. This benign lesion was first described by Dr. Donald Gass at Bascom Palmer Eye Institute in 1973 in seven patients. Although similar to an epiretinal membrane, it has a more striking funduscopic appearance.

64a. This painting demonstrates a juxtapapillary veneer of fibrous tissue that coalesces into a thickened epiretinal bulb of tissue just nasal to the fovea.

64b. This cross-sectional representation of the same patient demonstrates that the lesion is well away from the center of the fovea and does not cause distortion of the normal macular contour, with no macular edema or loss of the foveal depression.

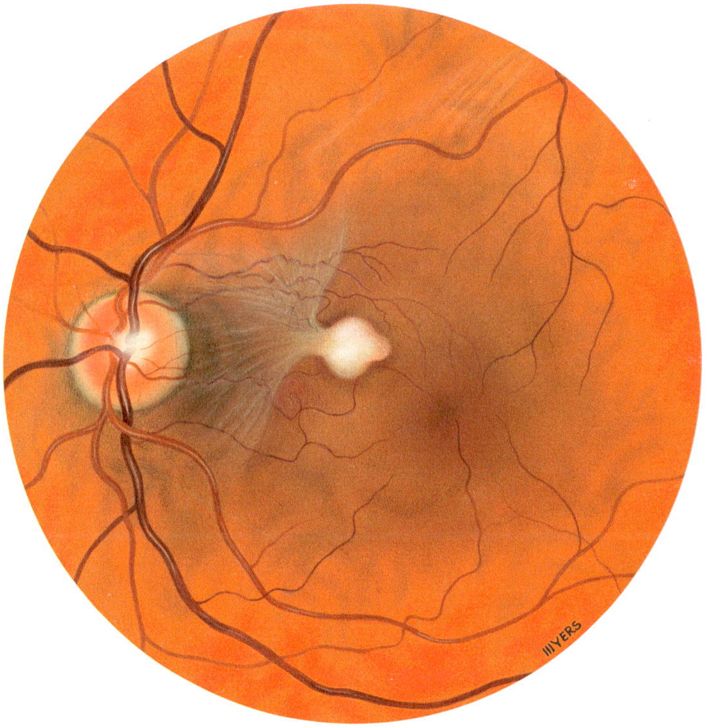

64a

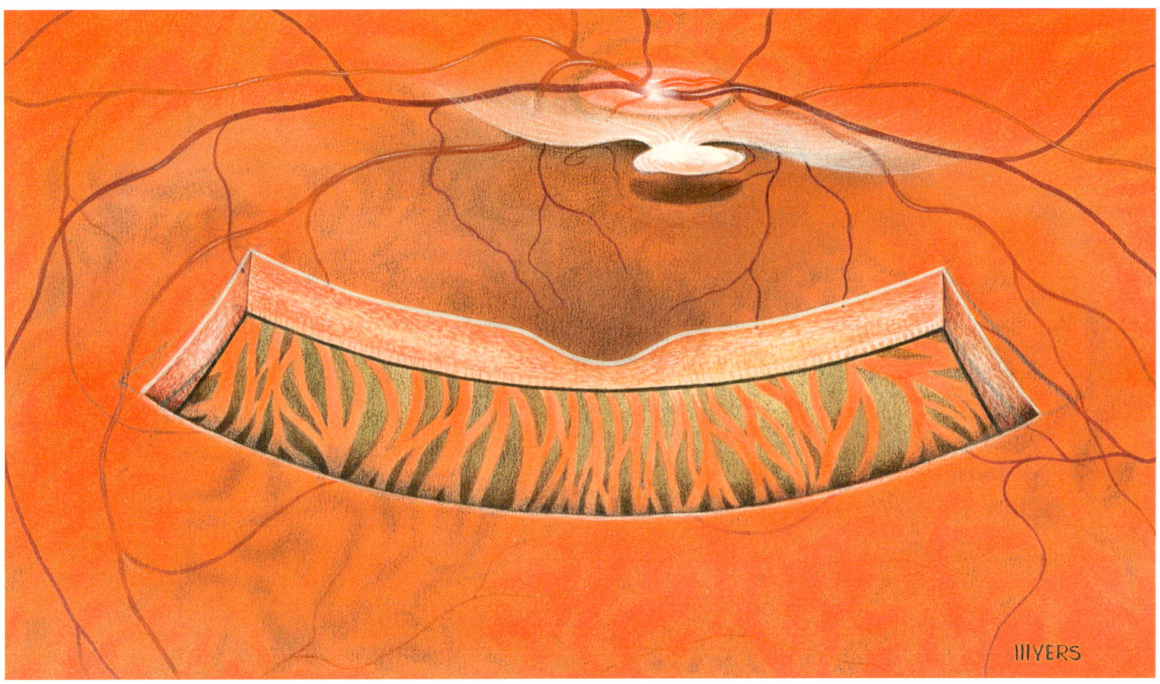

64b

PLATE 65

Idiopathic Full-Thickness Macular Hole

In these paintings, the patient has a full-thickness macular hole. A central defect in the macula is shown along with a persistent posterior hyaloid attachment. Dr. Gass at Bascom Palmer Eye Institute popularized the grading system of idiopathic full-thickness macular holes in several publications as well as in his classic textbook.

65a. This painting represents a patient with a Gass Stage II macular hole, insofar as a full-thickness defect is present along with incomplete separation of the vitreous with a hole that appears less than 400 microns in diameter.

65b. This painting represents a cross-sectional image of the same patient and demonstrates nicely how the vitreous is exerting traction on the inferior edge of the flap of the macular hole.

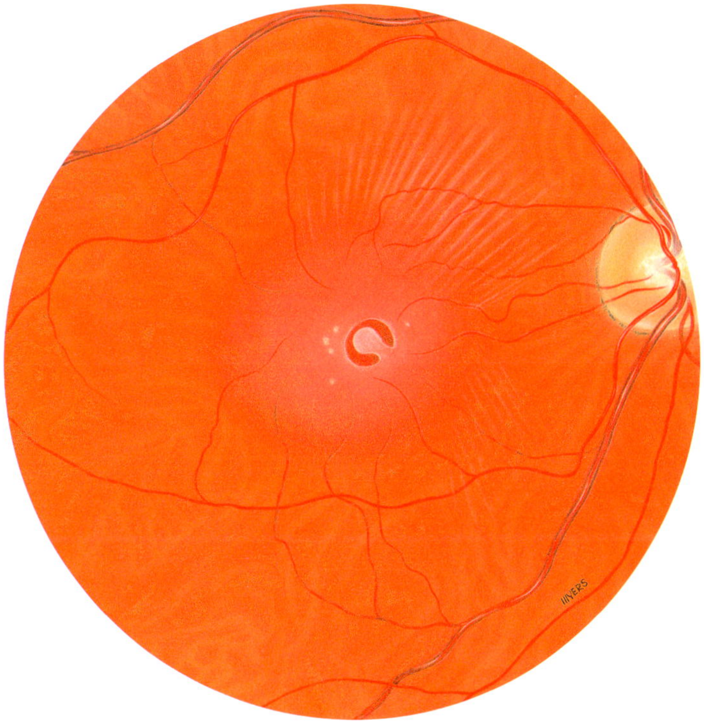

65a

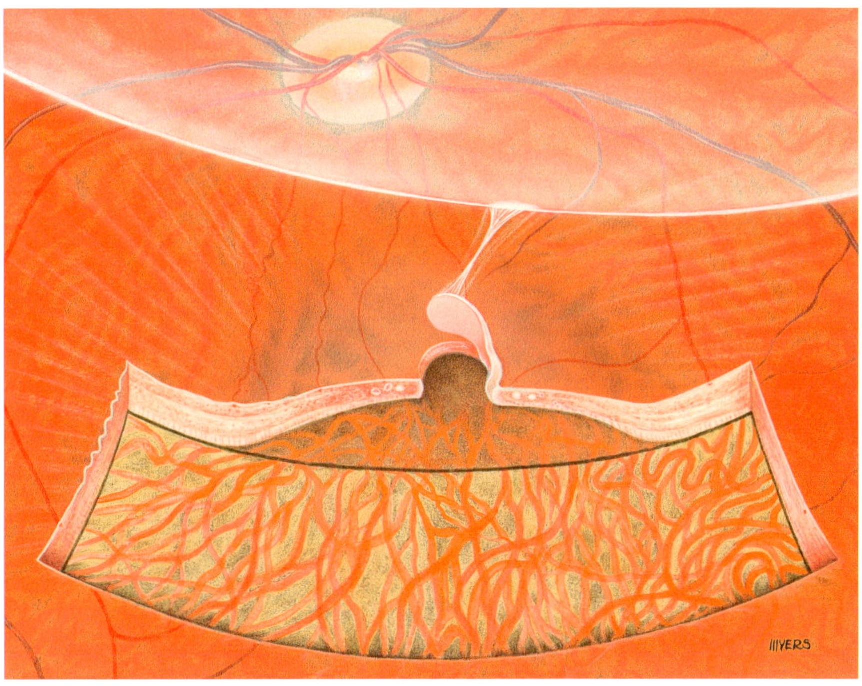

65b

PLATE 66

Posterior Vitreous Detachment

Posterior vitreous detachment occurs as the vitreous gel separates from the retinal surface, first at the top of the eye, then later in the back of the eye over the macula and around the optic nerve. Although posterior vitreous detachment is part of the normal aging process, the development of an acute and symptomatic posterior vitreous detachment is an urgent eye problem. Patients with an acute posterior vitreous detachment can observe an acute development of a visual opacity in their vision and are at risk for retinal tear or development of retinal detachment. This painting depicts a cross-sectional image of a posterior vitreous detachment that is more fully separated superiorly (left side of image) and remains attached at the fovea. The underlying retinal contour remains undisturbed.

(Paintings 62b, 63b and 66 were reproduced in black and white and published by Dr. Gass in: Gass JDM. Stereoscopic Atlas of Macular Disease; a Funduscopic and Angiographic Presentation, 1st ed. St. Louis, CV Mosby, 1970.)

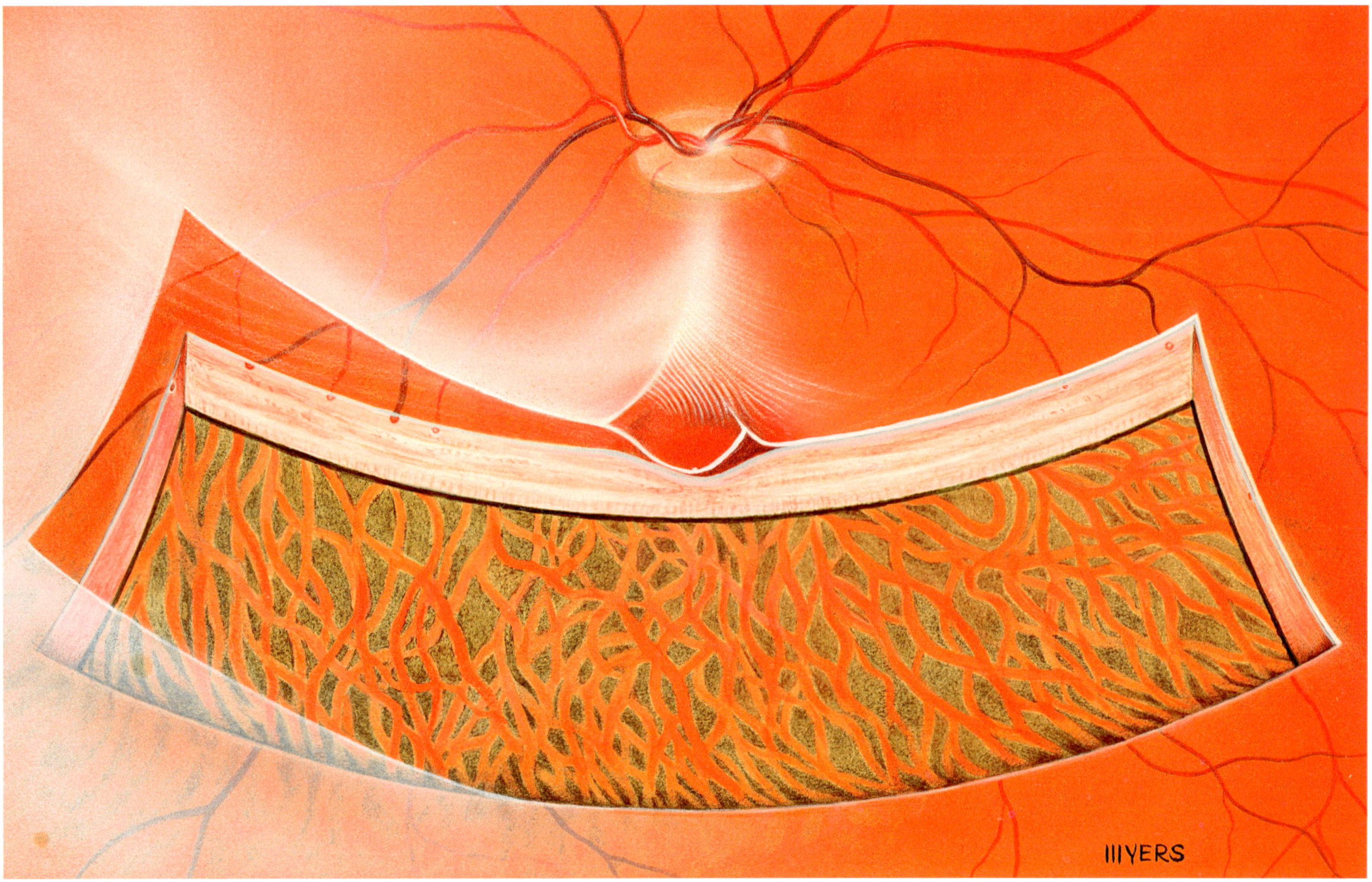

MYERS

PLATE 67

Vitreomacular Traction with Macular Edema

These patients have an abnormally adherent posterior vitreous face that remains broadly attached across the posterior pole and is exerting tractional forces on the macula that has developed macular edema as a result. Epiretinal membranes are commonly observed in this setting. This may resolve spontaneously or require surgical separation of the vitreous from the retinal surface.

67a. This painting depicts a cross-sectional image of a patient with vitreomacular traction and intraretinal fluid accumulation characterized by clearly delineated cystic spaces within the macula.

67b. This painting also depicts a cross-sectional image of a patient with vitreomacular traction and retinal edema with less well-delineated cystic spaces.

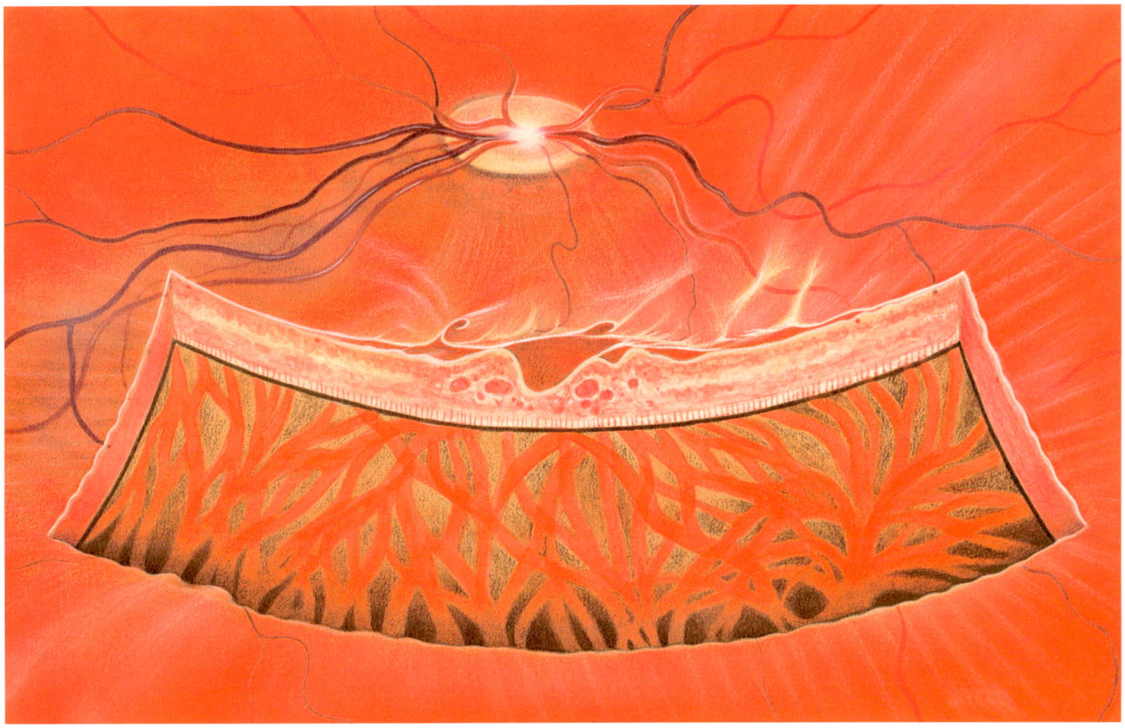

67a

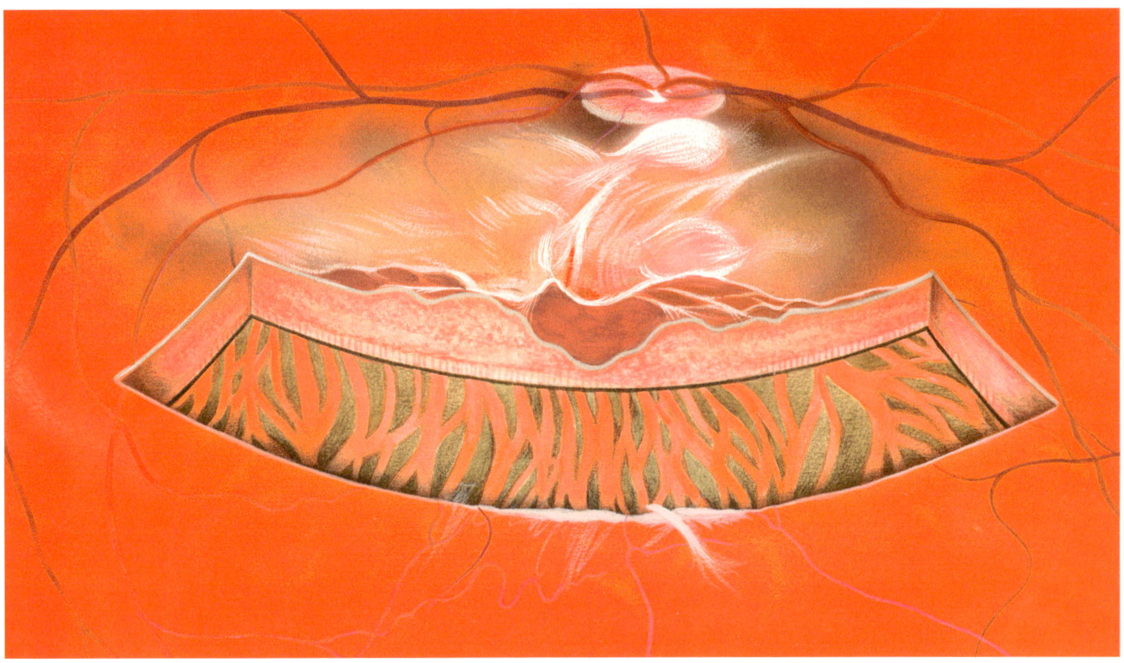

67b

PLATE 68

Retinal Fold and Epiretinal Membrane

These paintings represent patients with a surface proliferation consistent with an advanced epiretinal membrane, retinal edema and a retinal fold. These can be idiopathic, secondary to infectious or inflammatory conditions, or develop after repair of retinal detachment with a scleral buckle.

68a. The funduscopic appearance of a patient with profound surface proliferation of fibrous tissue, intraretinal hemorrhage and macular edema is illustrated in this painting.

68b. This painting also demonstrates a cross-sectional image of a patient with a retinal fold along the major venous arcade and underlying macular edema.

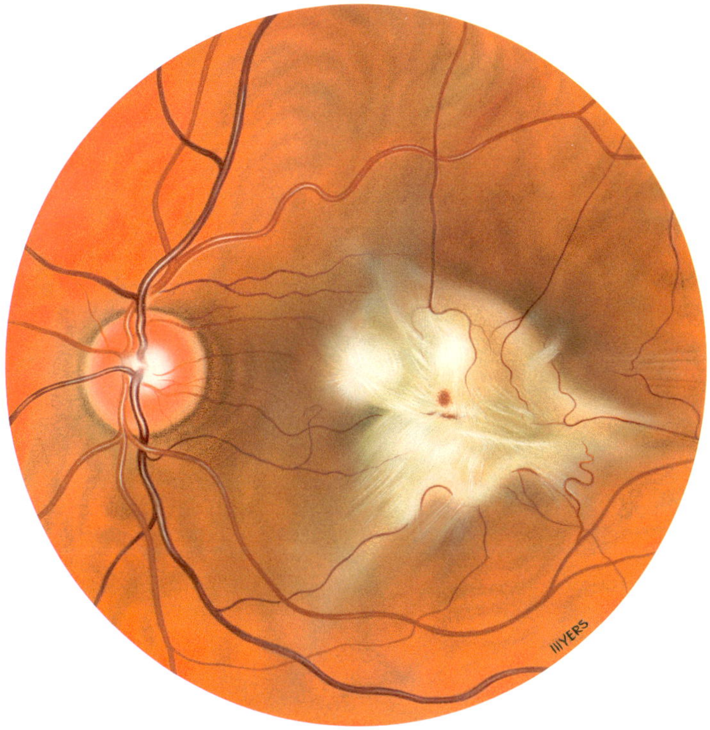

68a

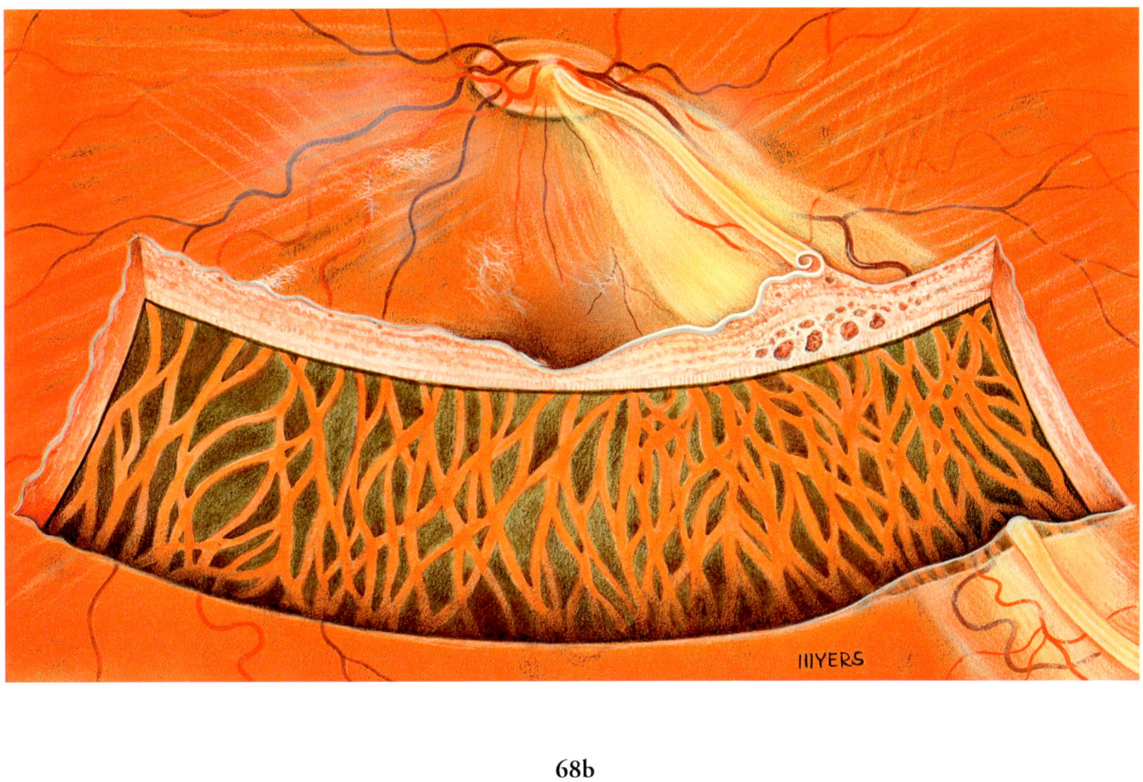

68b

PLATE 69

Idiopathic Full-Thickness Macular Hole

The Gass classification of idiopathic full-thickness macular holes differentiates between those patients with an attached hyaloid membrane (Gass Stage II) and a separated hyaloid membrane (Gass Stages III and IV). This painting demonstrates the cross-sectional appearance of a patient with an idiopathic full-thickness macular hole and attached hyaloid membranes and represents a Gass Stage II hole. Corrugations of the retina surface suggest an associated epiretinal membrane.

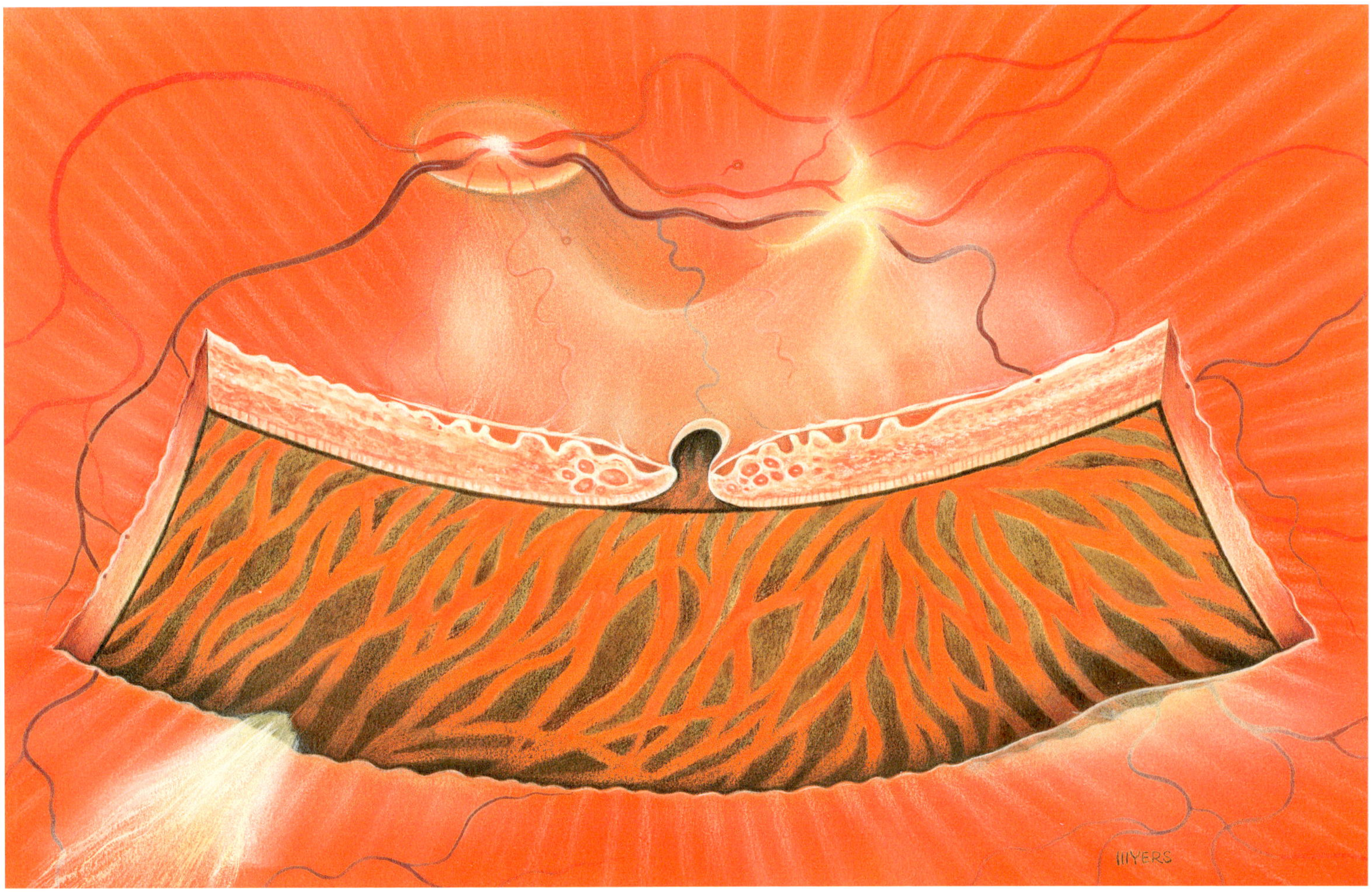
MYERS

PLATE 70

Bullous Retinoschisis

Patients with bullous retinoschisis have a split in the outer plexiform layer of the retina in a well-defined quadrant of the fundus. The involved area of retinoschisis corresponds to an absolute scotoma in a patient's visual field. This painting depicts a patient with a slit-lamp biomicroscopic fundus appearance of a localized area of bullous retinoschisis (bottom half of image) where the slit beams separate adjacent to an area of normal retina (top half of image) where the slit beams coalesce.

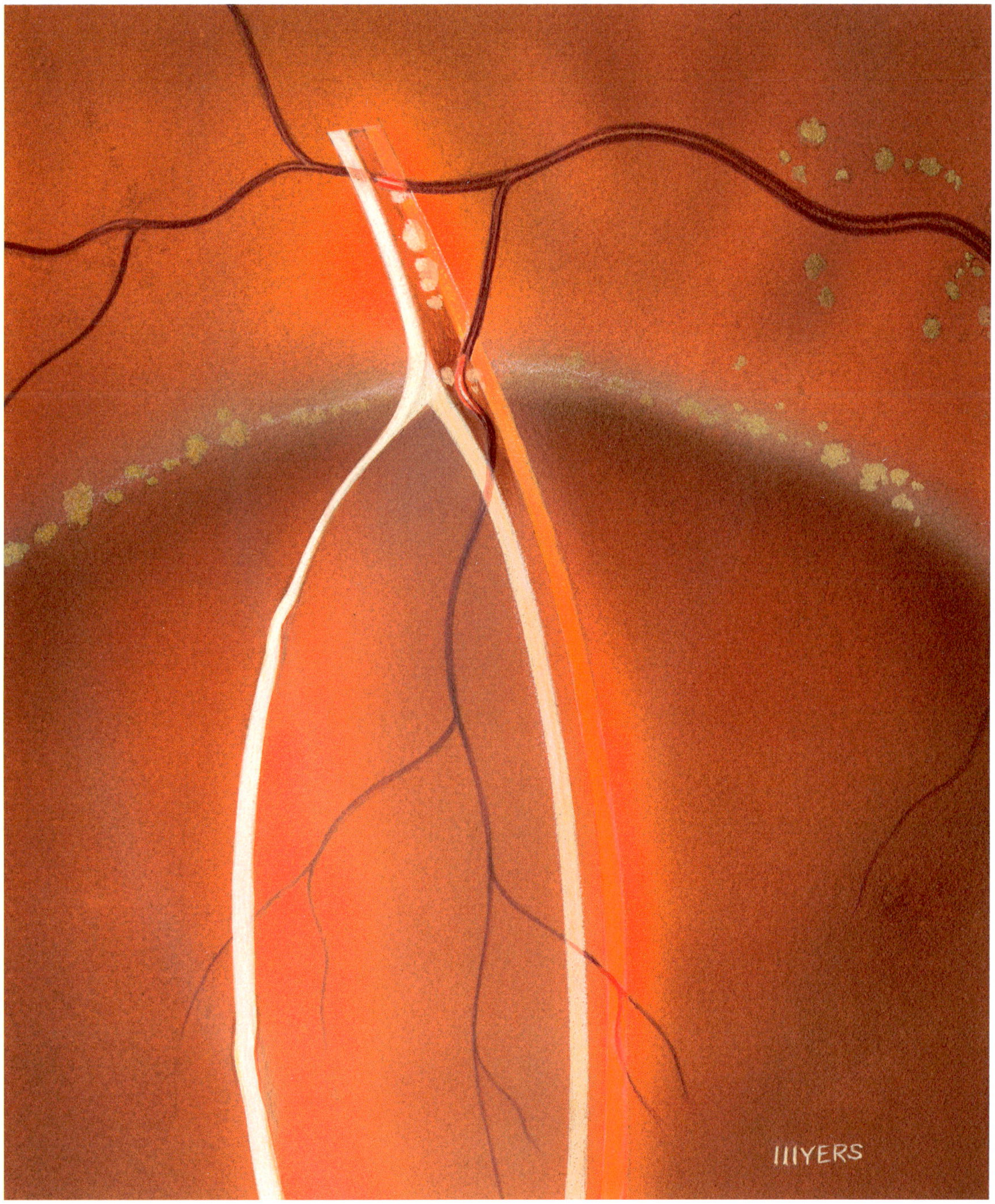
MYERS

PLATE 71

Branch Retinal Vein Occlusion and Retinal Edema

Retinal arteries and veins share a common adventitial sheath at crossing points. The weaker vein can become compressed by the stronger artery leading to arteriovenous nicking at one end of the spectrum and partial blockage of the retinal vein at the other. A branch retinal vein occlusion usually is associated with retinal hemorrhages and edema. This painting depicts the funduscopic appearance of a patient with a superotemporal branch retinal (tributary) vein occlusion with arteriovenous compression, venous engorgement and mild tortuosity, retinal flame-shaped and blot hemorrhages, exudates and edema. An associated mild epiretinal membrane is observed centrally.

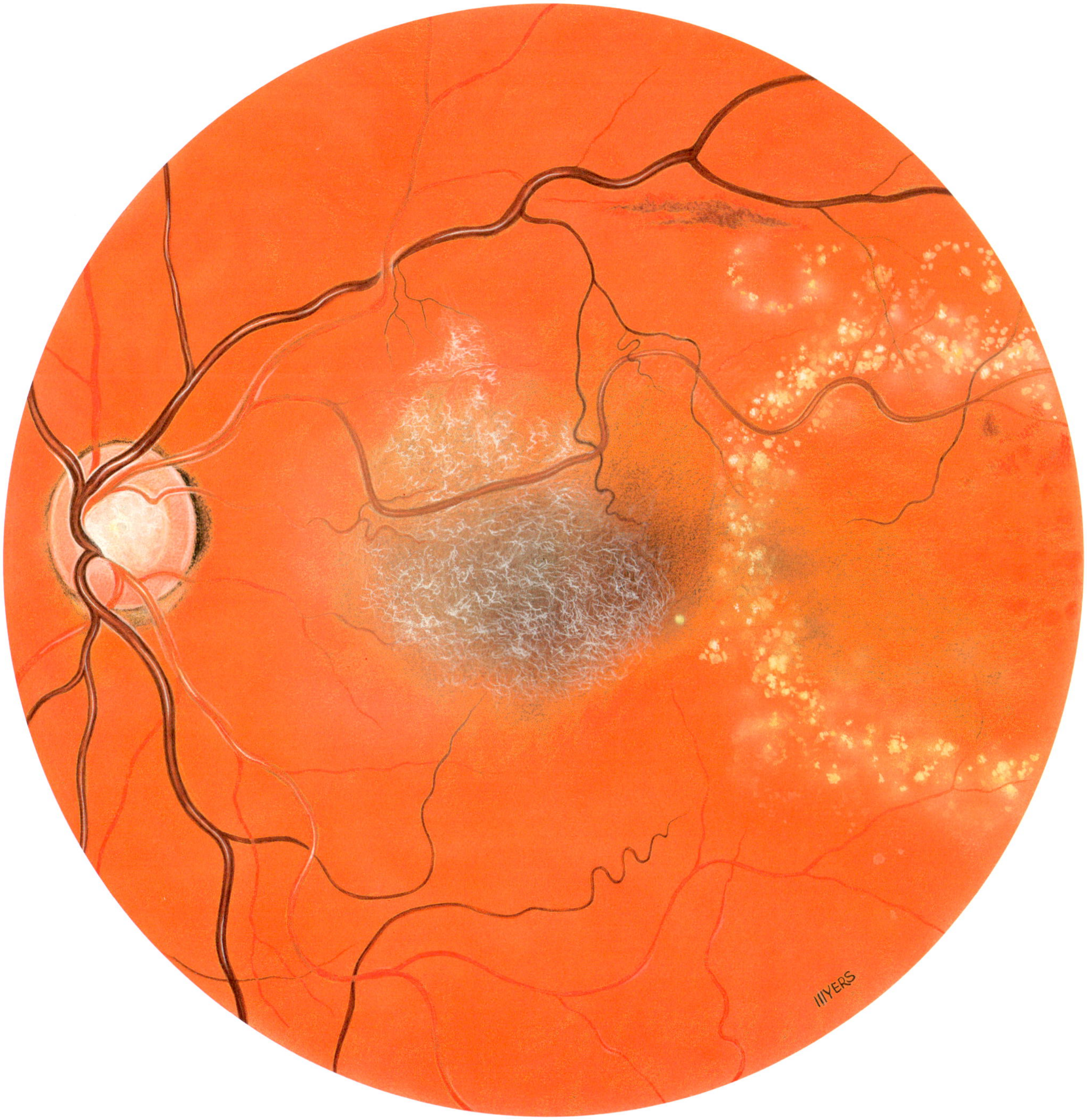

PLATE 72

Chronic Rhegmatogenous Retinal Detachment

Patients with a chronic retinal detachment secondary to peripheral retinal breaks can develop a stable or non-progressive appearance and become limited by a pigmented, so-called demarcation line. Additionally, patients can develop proliferative vitreoretinopathy represented by pigmented cells in the vitreous and contractile membranes on the retinal surfaces. This painting demonstrates the ophthalmoscopic appearance of a patient with a chronic rhegmatogenous retinal detachment with atrophic retinal holes, surface proliferative vitreoretinopathy and a demarcation line.

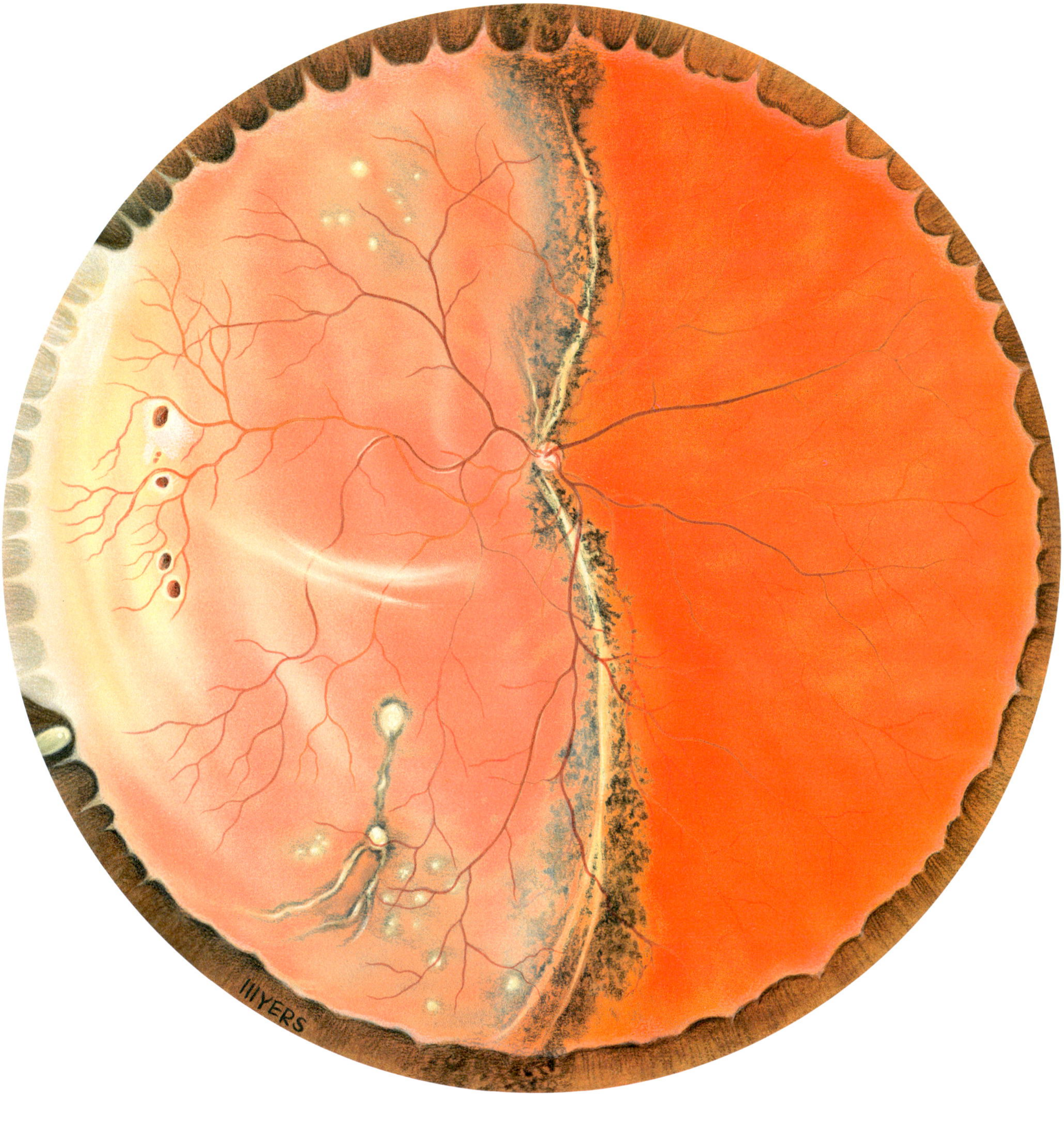
MYERS

PLATE 73

Proliferative Vitreoretinopathy-Related Retinal Detachment

Advanced proliferative vitreoretinopathy from rhegmatogenous retinal detachment can result in fixed retinal folds, fibrotic star folds, preretinal and subretinal fibrotic bands and stiffened retina. It is the number one cause of a failed retinal detachment repair. This painting illustrates the funduscopic appearance of a patient with a total rhegmatogenous retinal detachment with multiple star-fold figures, multiple retinal breaks and disorganized retina.

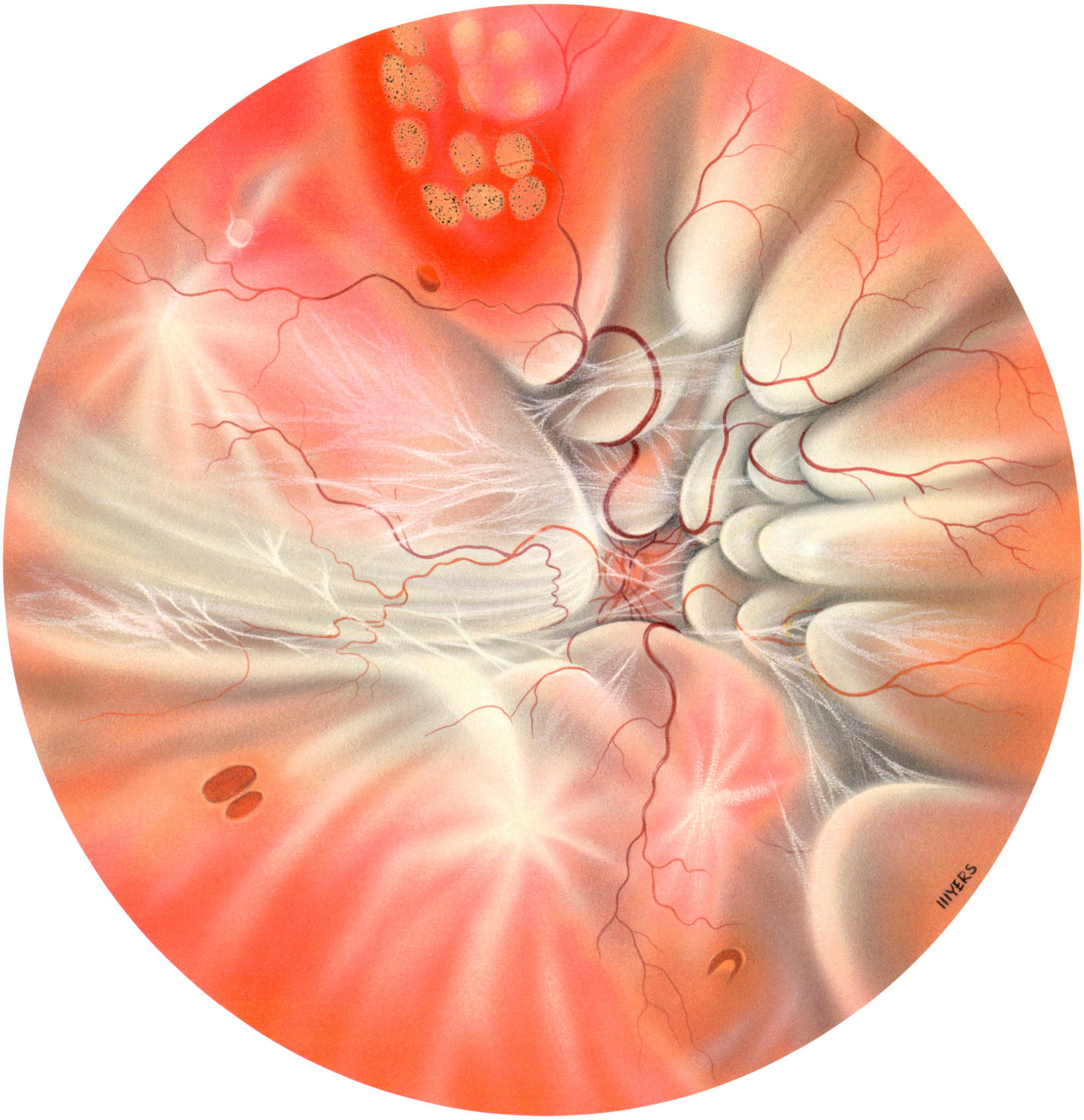
MYERS

PLATE 74

Pigmented Fundus Lesion

There are a variety of pigmented fundus lesions that require close scrutiny. Most of these are benign, but the specter of posterior uveal malignant melanoma or metastases must always be kept in mind. This painting represents an elevated peripheral pigmented fundus lesion and associated satellite lesions that extend to the ora serrata and circumferentially. Morphologically, this appears to have grapelike clusters and is consistent with a benign cavernous retinal hemangioma.

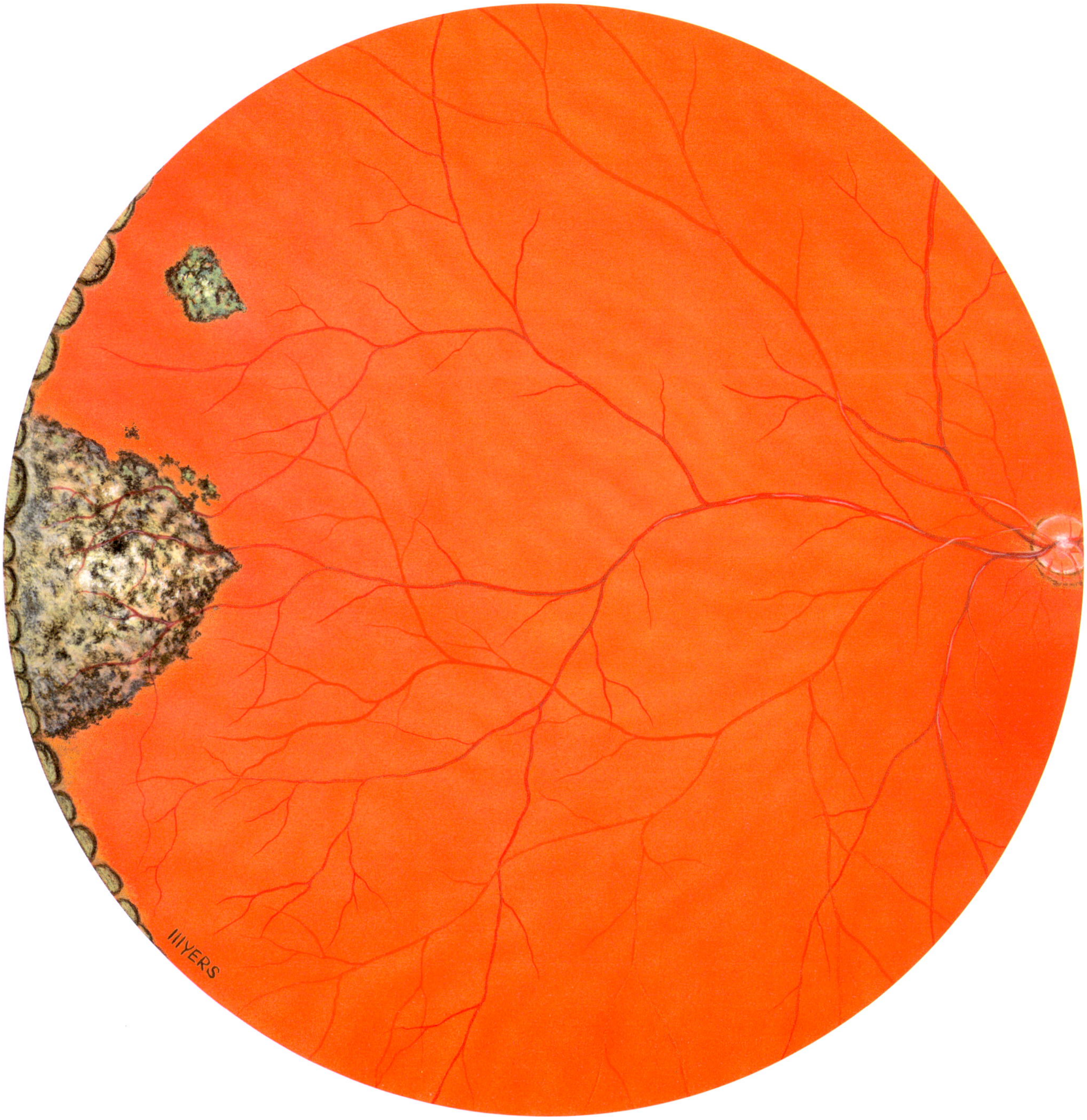

PLATE 75

Elevated Fundus Mass

There are also a variety of non-pigmented fundus masses that require close scrutiny. One should always be vigilant for an amelanotic melanoma or a metastatic lesion in an adult and a retinoblastoma in an infant or toddler. This painting represents a large peripheral fundus mass feeding and draining arteries and veins, an exudative retinal detachment and surface hemorrhages.

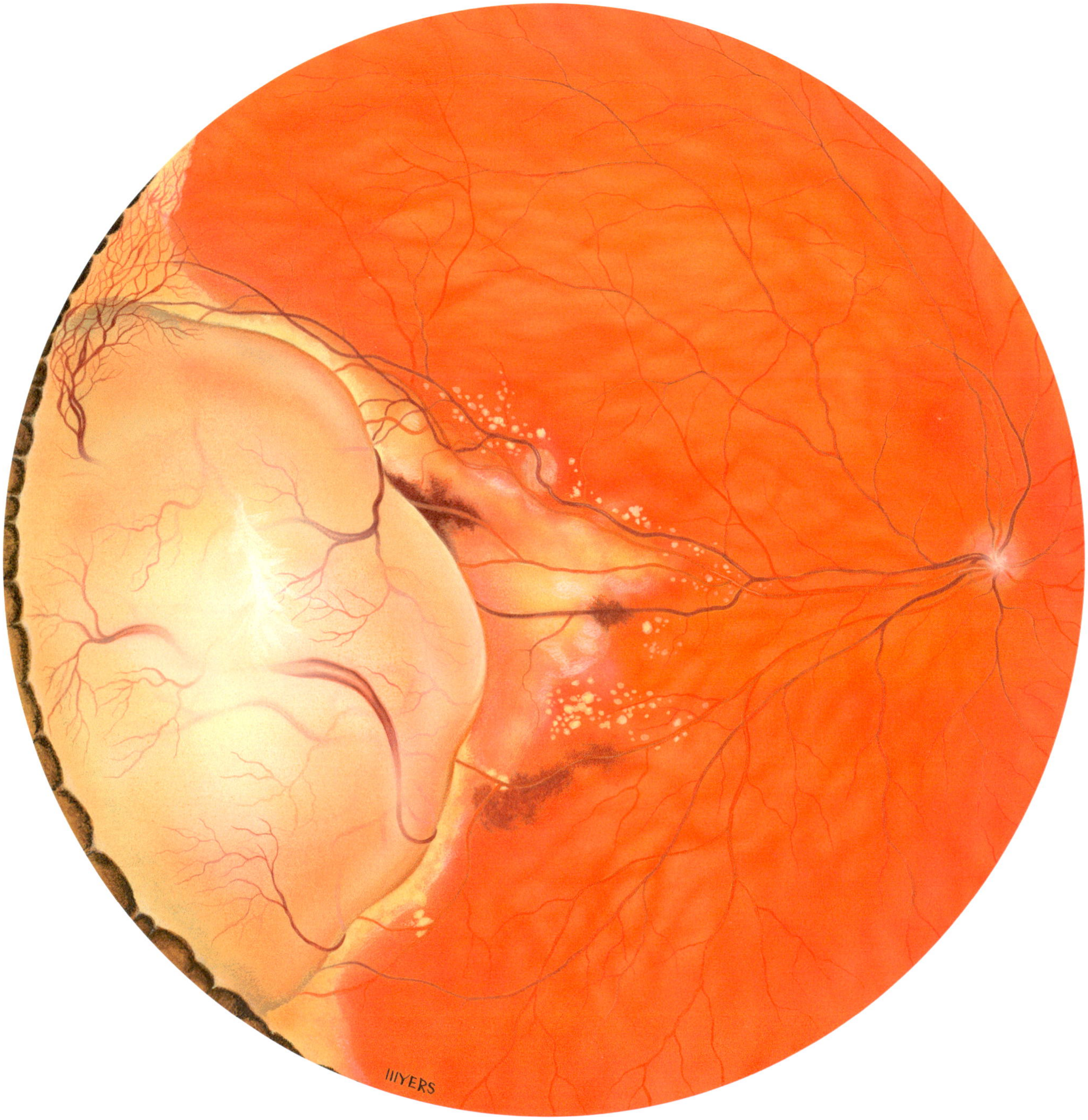
MYERS

PLATE 76

Diabetic Retinopathy

Loss of the integrity of the inner blood–retinal barrier (the tight junctions of the retinal vascular endothelium) typically seen in diabetic retinopathy, can lead to leakage of serum, lipid and whole blood from the vascular channels into the retinal layers. The ophthalmoscopic image in this painting depicts retinal vascular leakage leading to macular edema, accumulation of lipids in the macula and intraretinal hemorrhages. Well-circumscribed pale white lesions along the major vessels are most consistent with retinal xenon-arc photocoagulation, previously used to treat diabetic retinopathy.

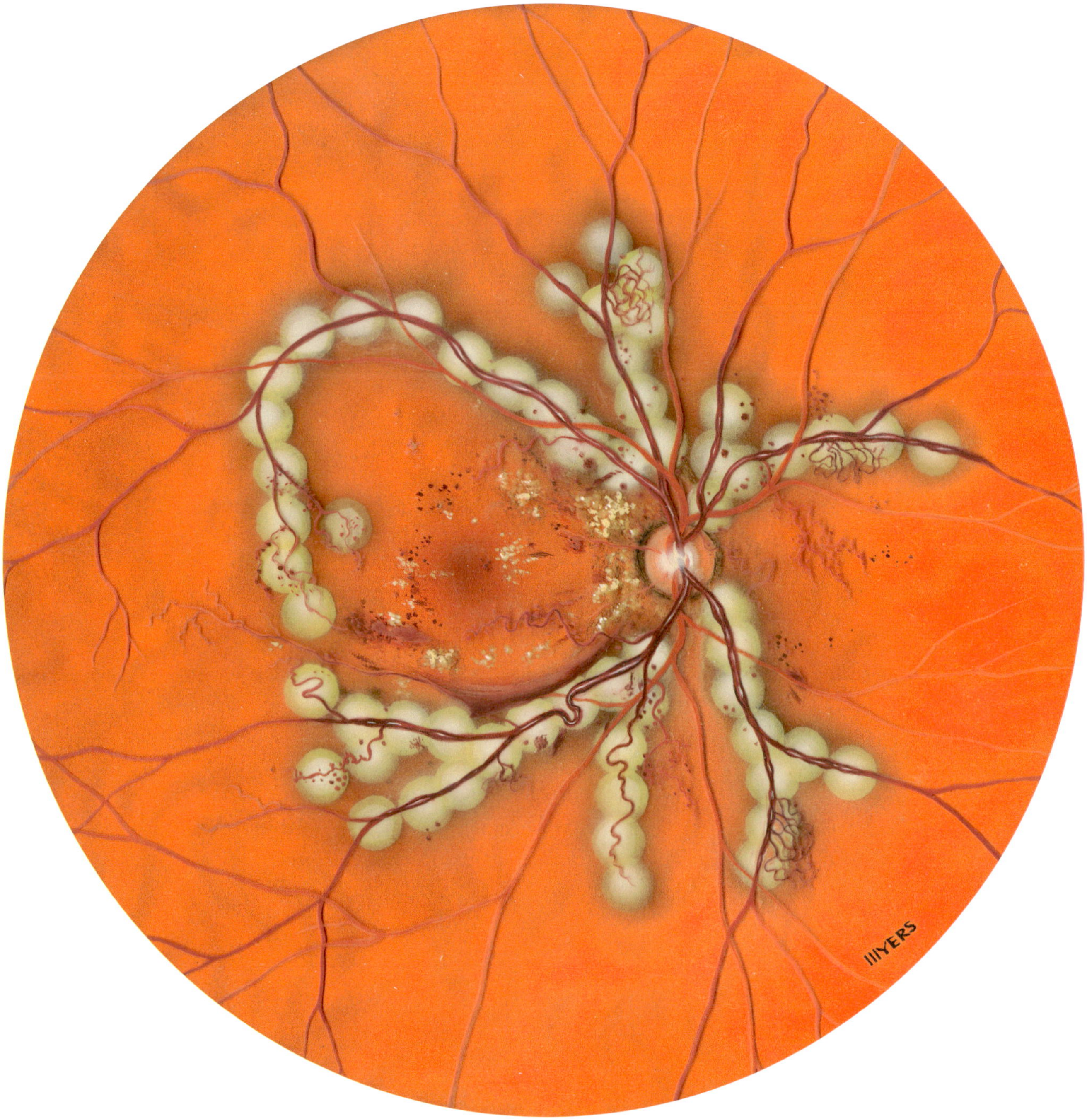
MYERS

PLATE 77

Elevated Fundus Mass

There are also a variety of non-pigmented fundus masses that require close observation and evaluation. As with the lesion in Plate 75, consideration of an amelanotic melanoma or metastatic lesion in an adult and a retinoblastoma in a child should be considered in the differential diagnosis. Vascular lesions like Coats disease can also present with a similar lesion. The image in this painting is consistent with Coats disease with a characteristic peripheral exudative retinal detachment and superficial retinal telangiectasia.

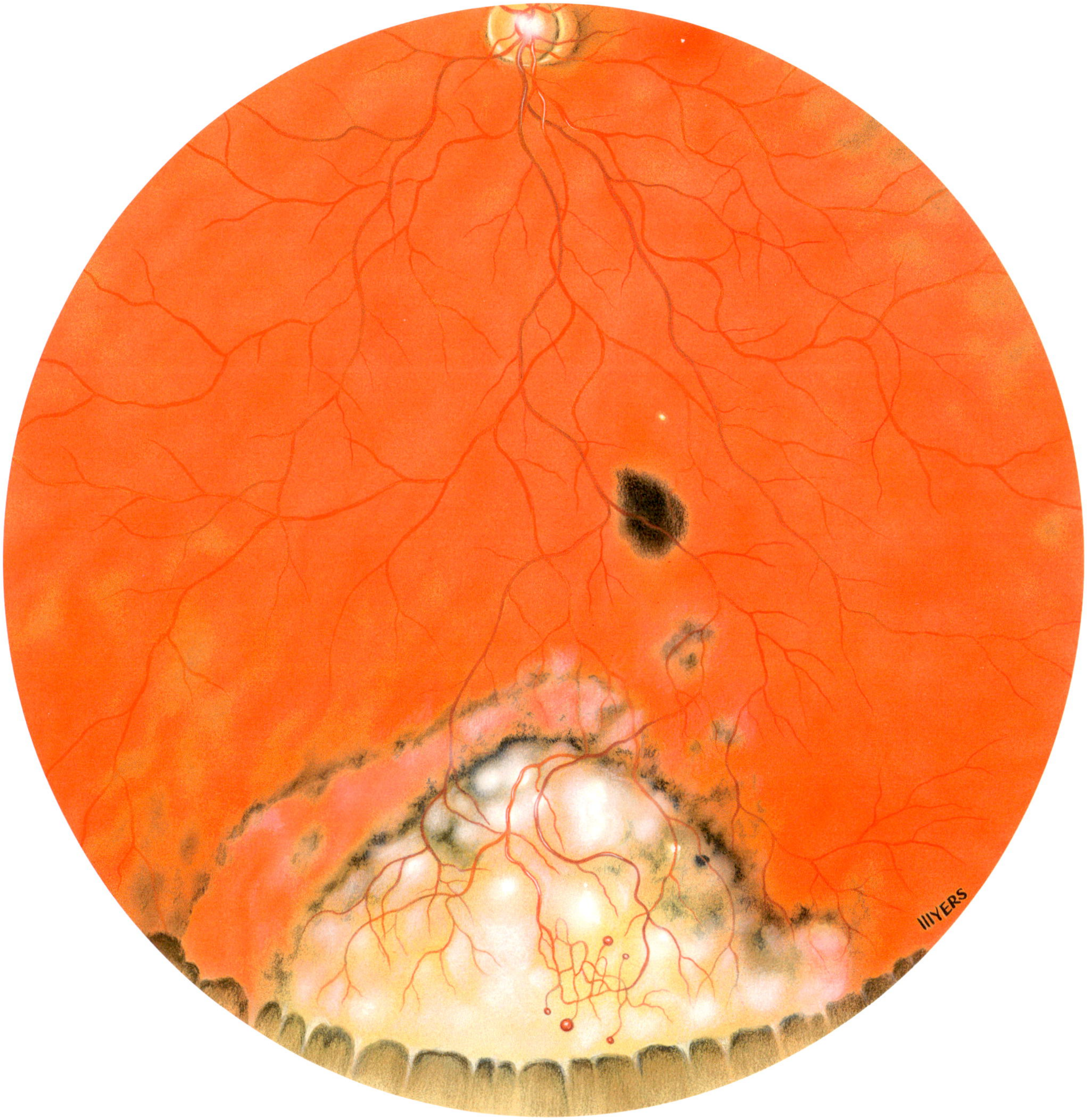
MYERS

PLATE 78

Coats Disease

Non-rhegmatogenous retinal detachment secondary to excessive capillary leakage from hyperpermeable retinal telangiectases is common in Coats disease, which is a unilateral disease typically affecting young boys and can often be confused with a lethal retinoblastoma. This painting represents a patient who has a peripheral exudative retinal detachment, surrounding retinal lipid exudates and peripheral telangiectactic vascular abnormalities.

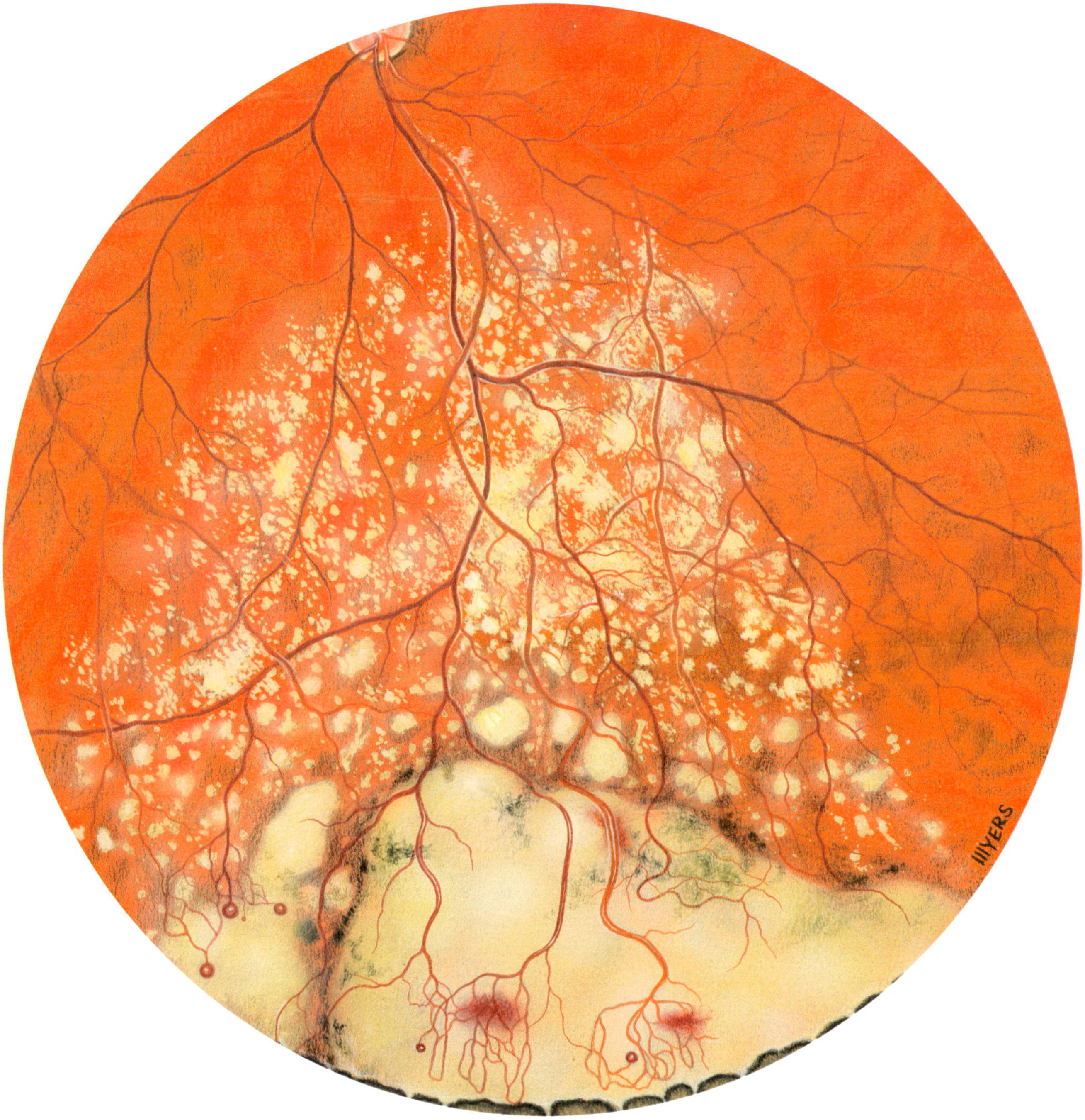

PLATE 79

Central Areolar Choroidal Dystrophy

Geographic atrophy of the macula refers to slowly expanding zones of devitalized retina and retinal pigment epithelium. Although seen most commonly in age-related macular degeneration, this type of retinal atrophy can be seen in the very rare central areolar choroidal dystrophy, as well as in numerous retinal inflammatory and degenerative diseases. The funduscopic image in this painting demonstrates large areas of geographic atrophy in a circumpapillary, macular and peripheral retinal configuration that is consistent with central areolar choroidal dystrophy.

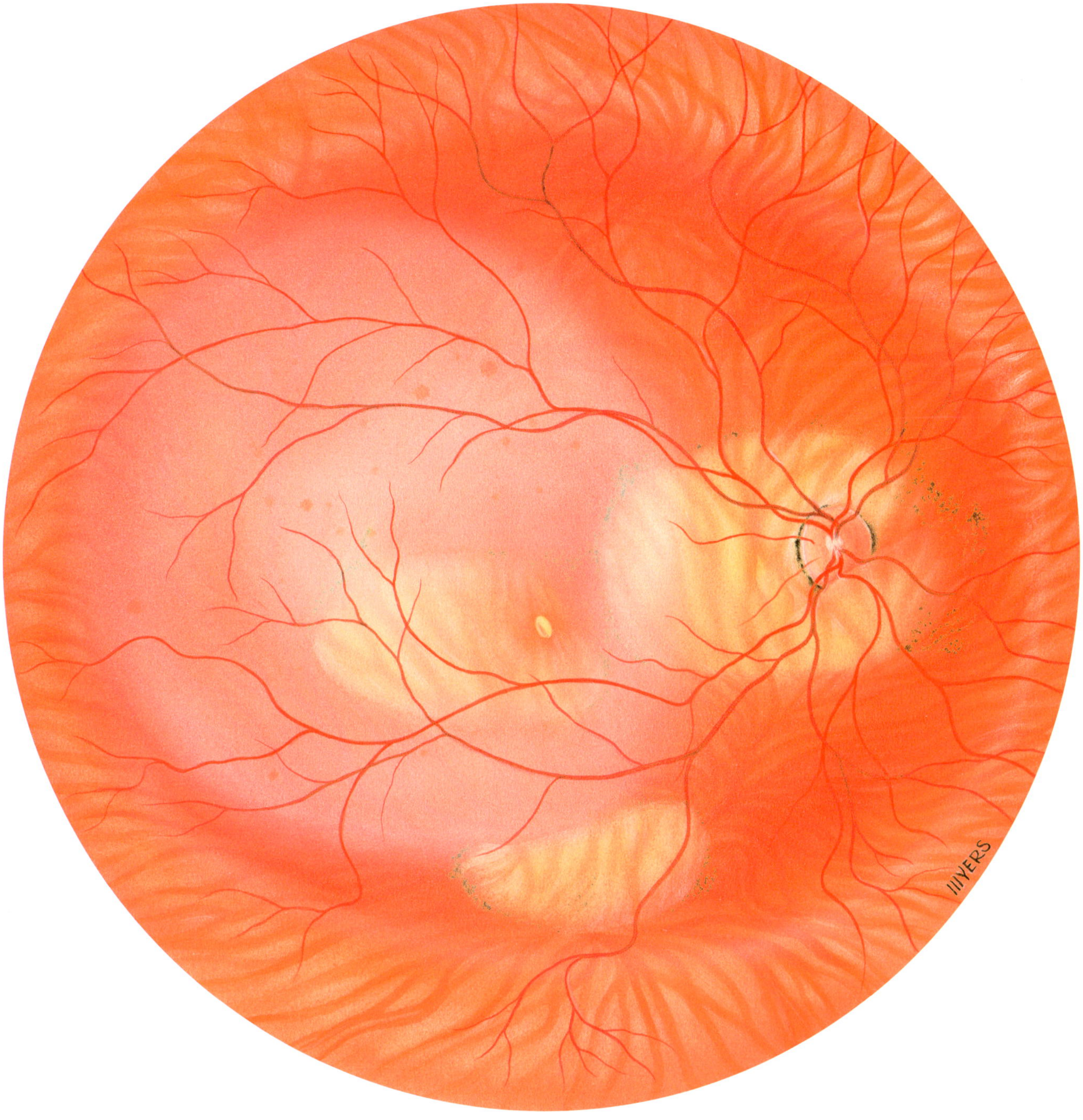

PLATE 80

Giant Retinal Tear

Rhegmatogenous retinal detachment is typically the result of a small- or medium-sized peripheral retinal break. Uncommonly, a patient can present with a retinal detachment secondary to a giant retinal tear that extends for three or more circumferential clock hours and can cause the retina to fold backward upon itself. The funduscopic appearance of a giant retinal tear-associated rhegmatogenous retinal detachment is depicted in this painting.

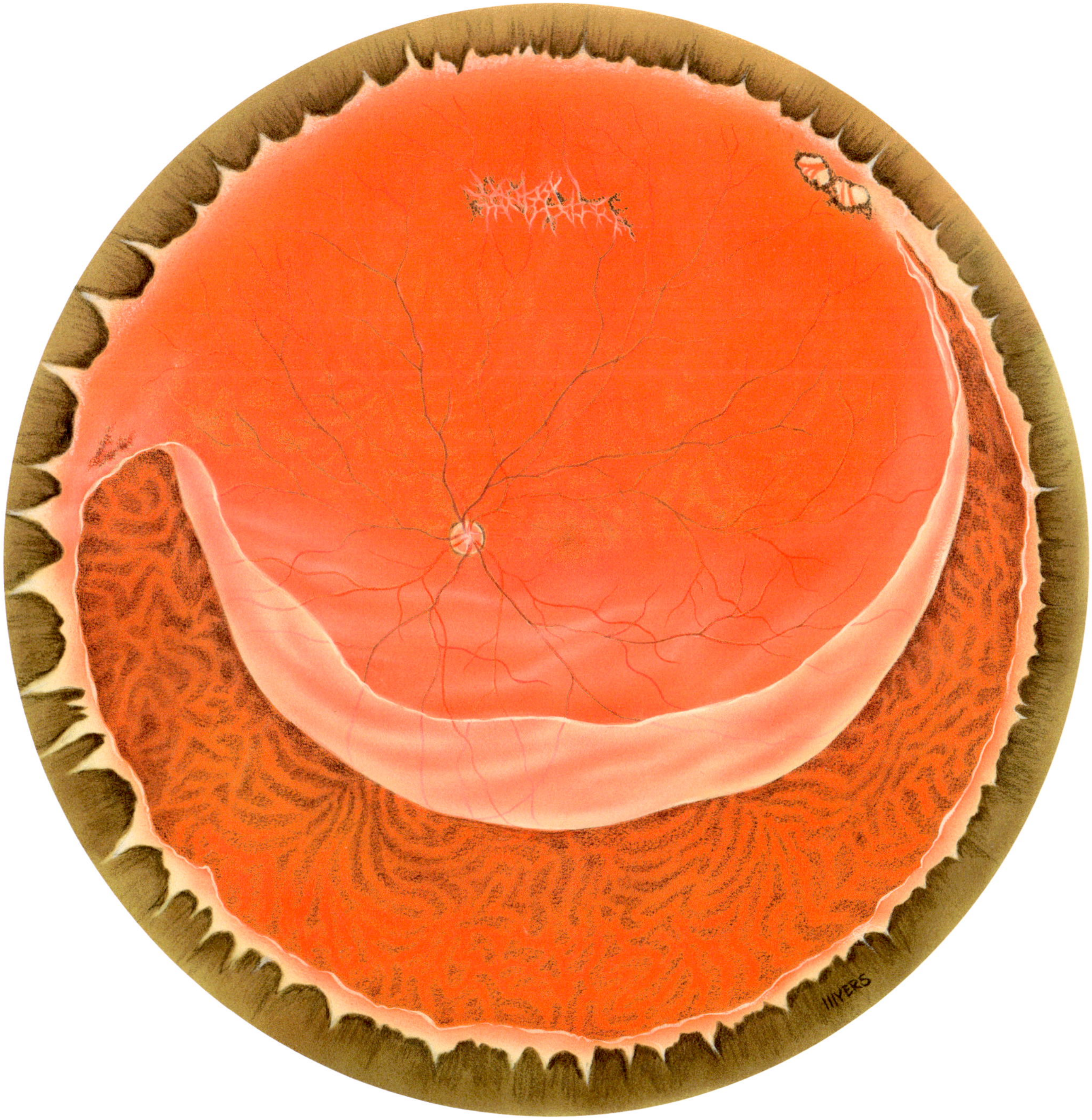
MYERS

PLATE 82

Pigmentary Retinopathy and Pigmented Fundus Mass

When the retinal pigment epithelium is disturbed, inflamed or traumatized, it can migrate anteriorly and deposit itself in the overlying retina in a spiculated pattern. This is seen most commonly in retinitis pigmentosa, but can also be observed in eyes with chronic inflammation, in eyes that suffered blunt trauma and in choroidal melanoma. This painting depicts the funduscopic appearance of diffuse pigment deposition and a peripheral malignant melanoma arising from the ciliary body.

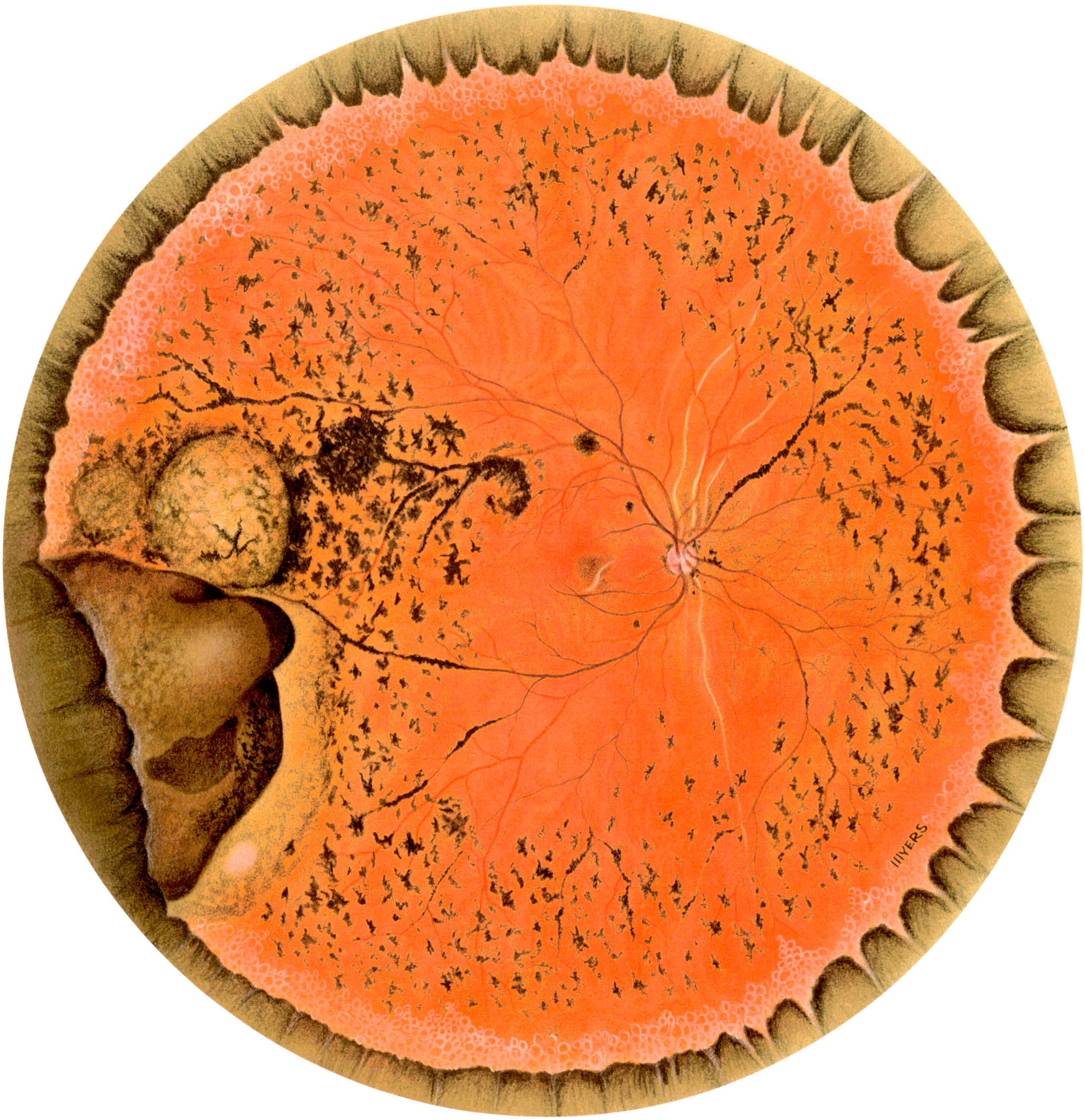
MYERS

PLATE 83

Malignant Choroidal Melanoma with Pigmentary Retinopathy

This is a high-magnification painting of the same patient in Plate 82, with the anteriorly located melanoma appearing as a silhouette. This painting demonstrates the appearance of the peripheral darkly pigmented lesion next to an area of adjacent retinal cysts in the setting of diffuse pigment hyperplasia.

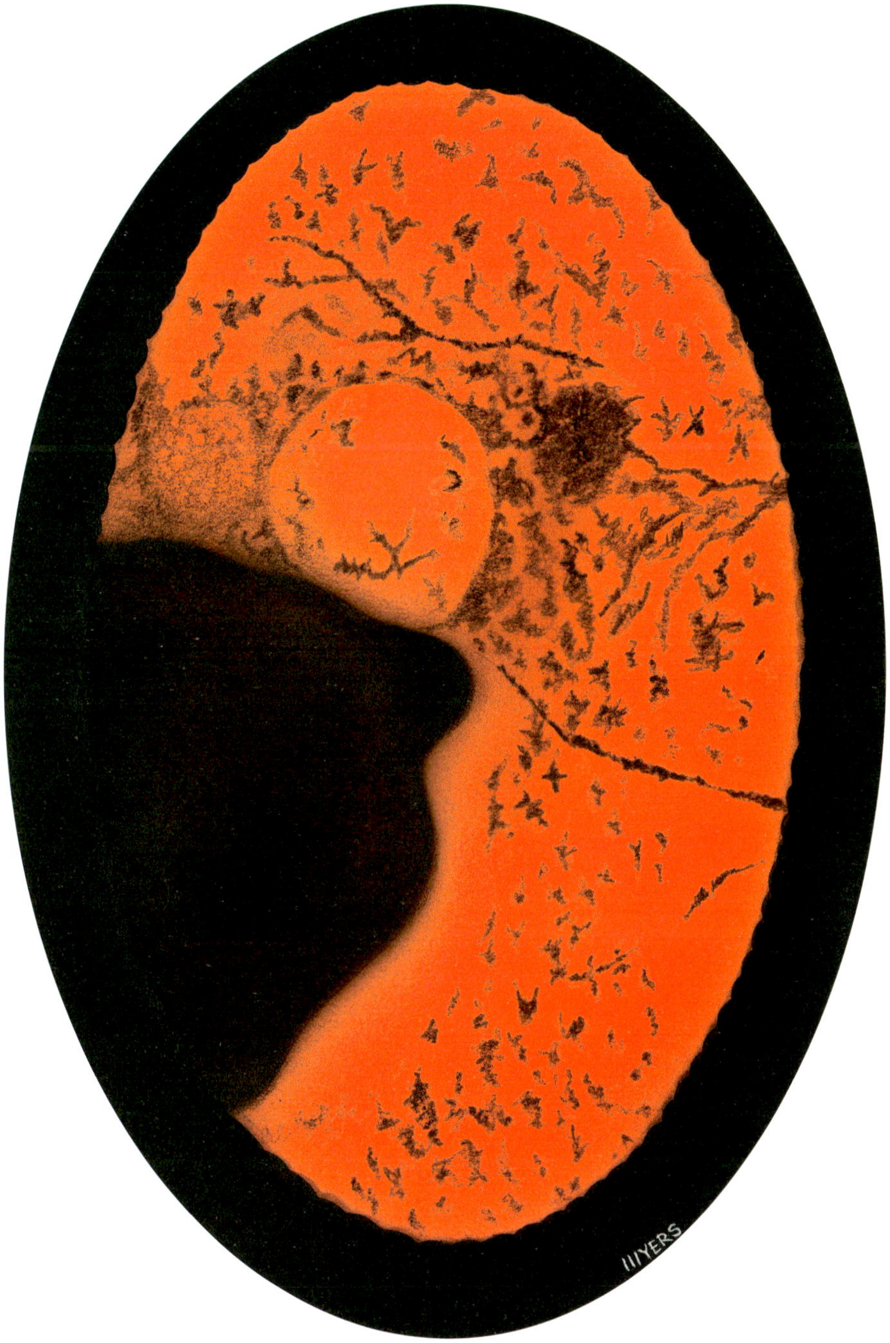

PLATE 84

Pigmented Fundus Lesion and Serous Retinal Detachment

A well-circumscribed pigmented fundus lesion is depicted with surrounding, probably serous, retinal detachment. The ophthalmoscopic appearance of a well-demarcated pigmented peripheral retinal lesion is consistent with hypertrophy of the retinal pigment epithelial lesion with diffuse serous retinal detachment.

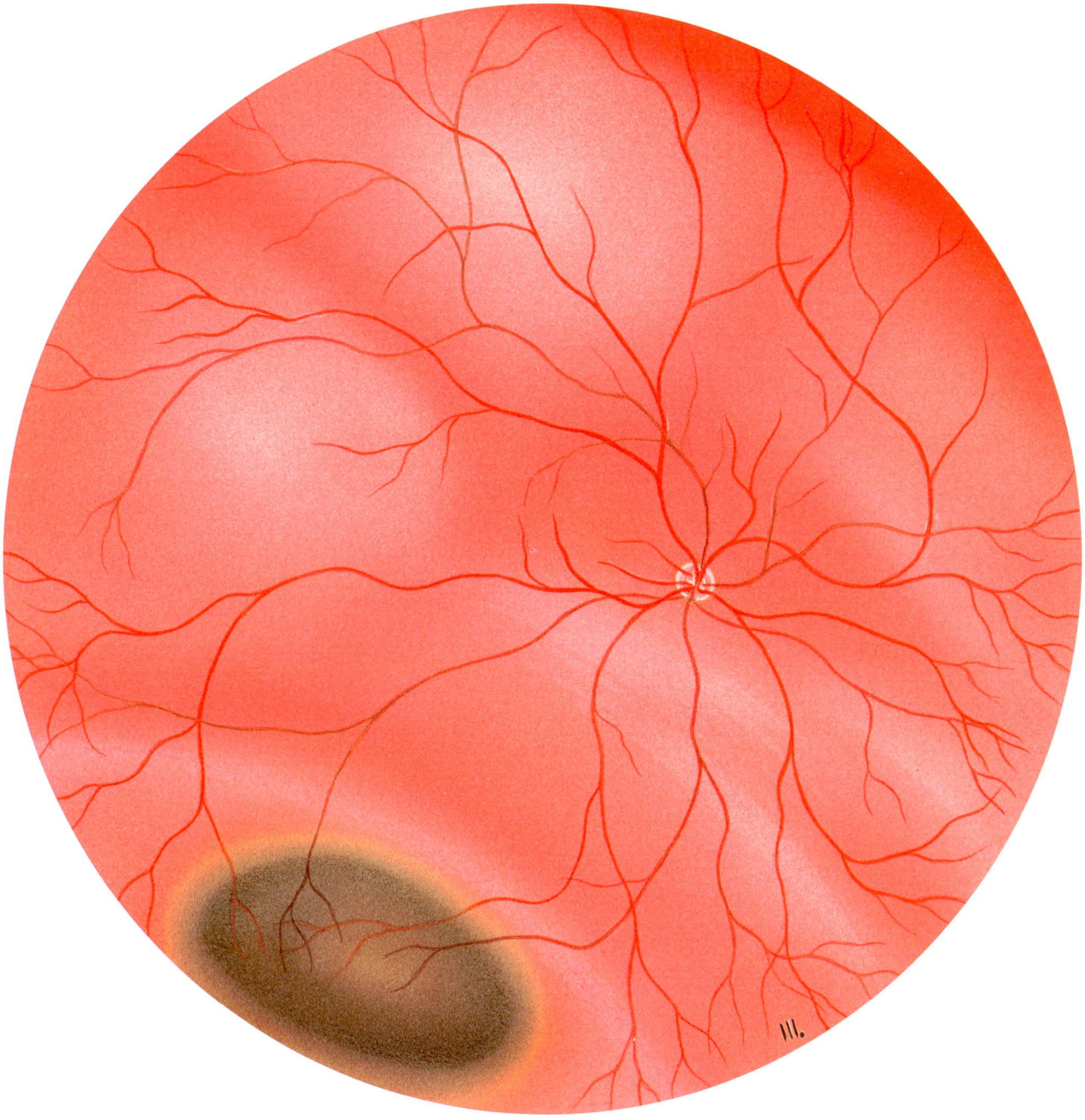

PLATE 85

Serous Retinal Detachment

Retinal detachments due to exudative processes (vascular or inflammatory causes) demonstrate shifting of subretinal fluid with changing body positions. Retinal detachments secondary to traction or peripheral retinal breaks do not manifest such shifting fluid. This painting demonstrates a retinal detachment with no peripheral retinal breaks or traction. Two distinct elevated areas of retina suggest a serous or exudative retinal detachment that may shift in configuration with changing body position.

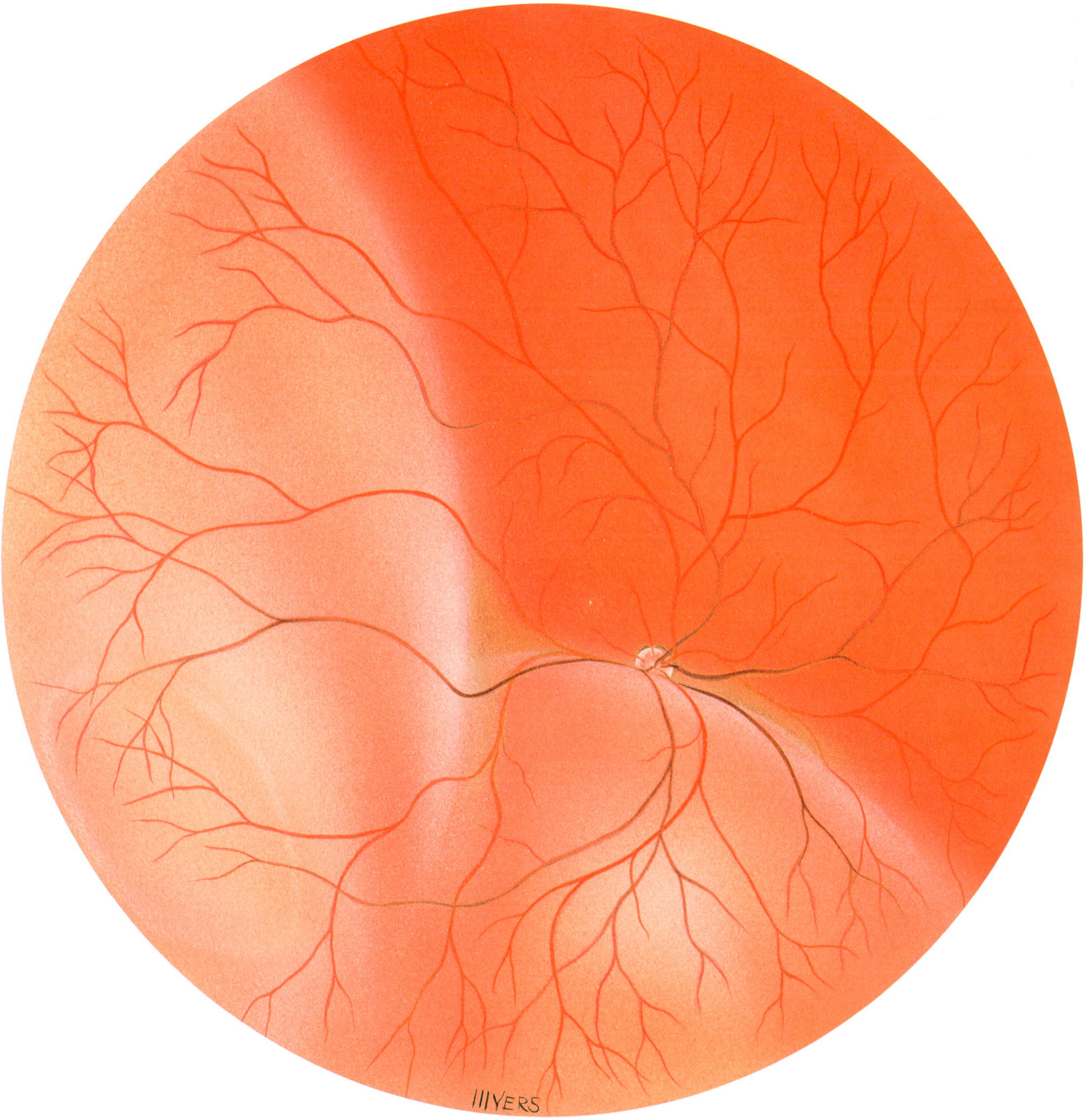
MYERS

PLATE 86

Choroidal Effusion or Detachment

The choroidal layer under the retina can become engorged during periods of low intraocular pressure or as a result of ocular inflammation. This is also referred to as choroidal detachment and may be serous or hemorrhagic in nature. This black and white painting was the last produced by Mr. Myers in August 1968, shortly before his final illness. It demonstrates the ophthalmoscopic appearance of a patient with shallow areas of peripheral serous choroidal effusions.

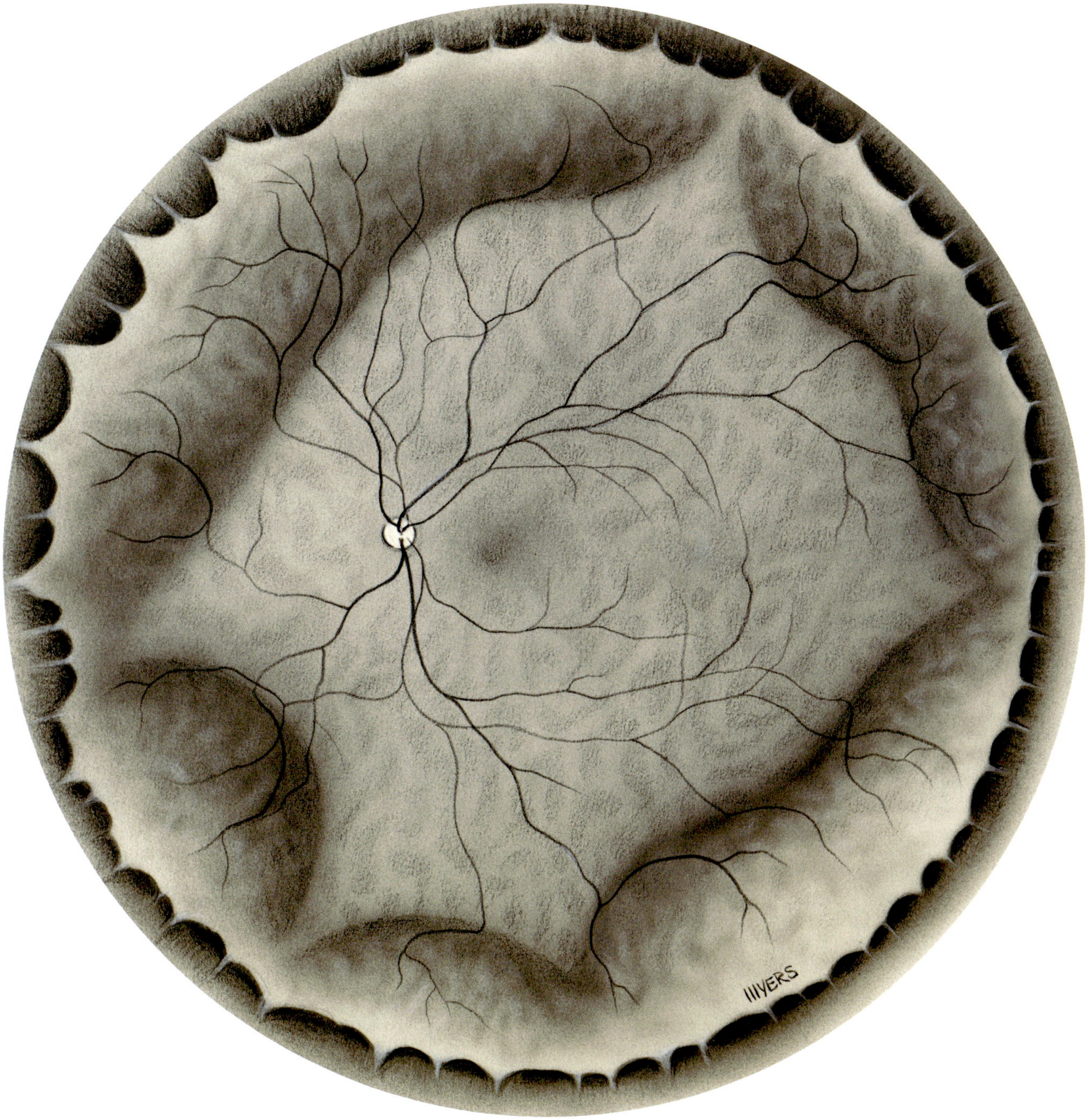
MYERS

PLATE 87a–d

Scleral Buckling Techniques

Grayscale illustrations of localized scleral buckling procedure techniques for repair of retinal holes with detachments.

a–d: Segmental Buckle for Repair of Retinal Hole

a: Identification and marking of equatorial retinal hole.
b: Segmental equatorial buckle.
c: Segmental equatorial buckle placed under superior rectus muscle.
d: Radial placement of scleral buckle for larger retinal hole requiring removal of rectus muscle, placement of buckle and resuturing of muscle.

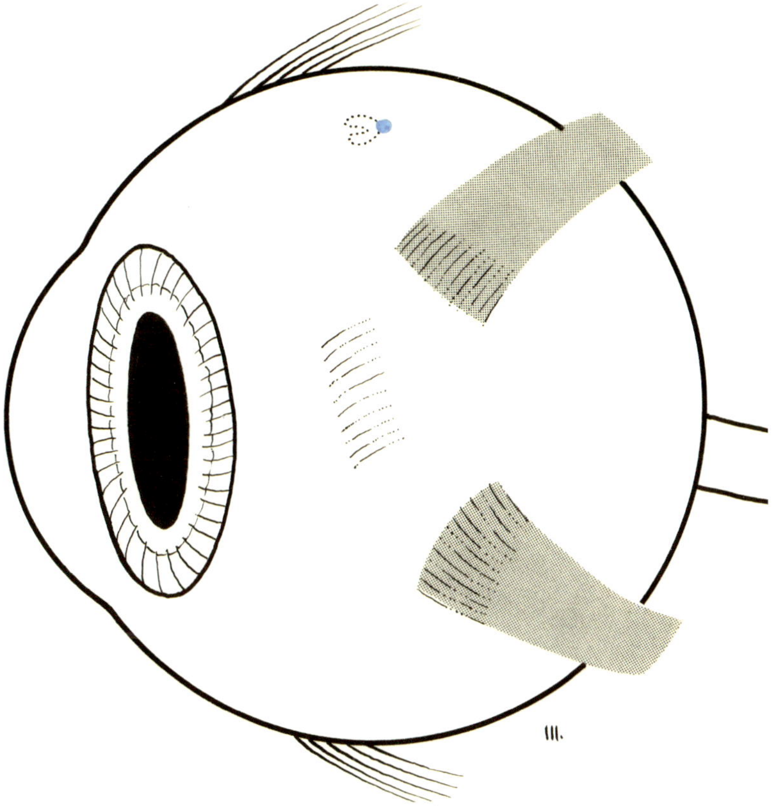

87a

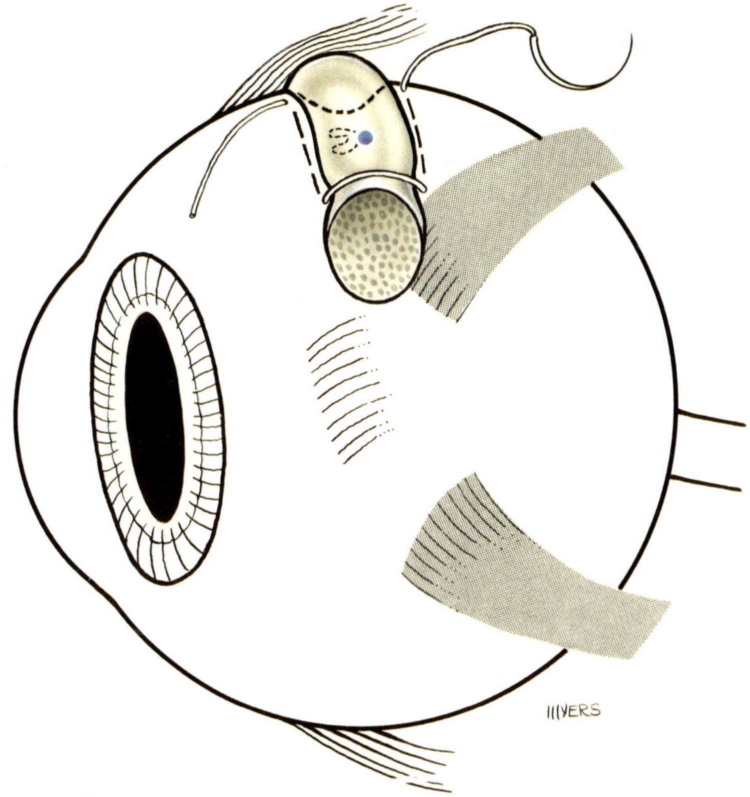

87b

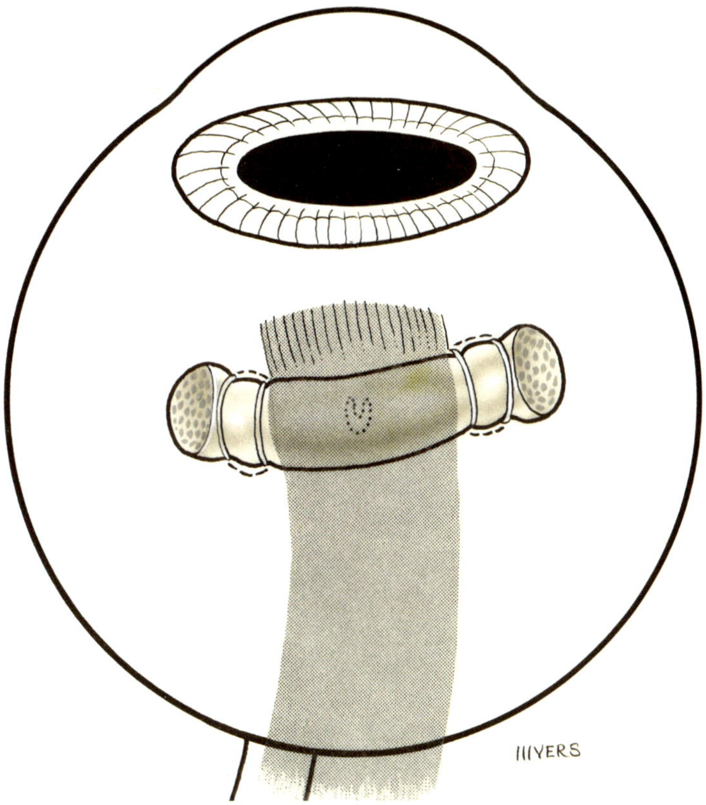

87c

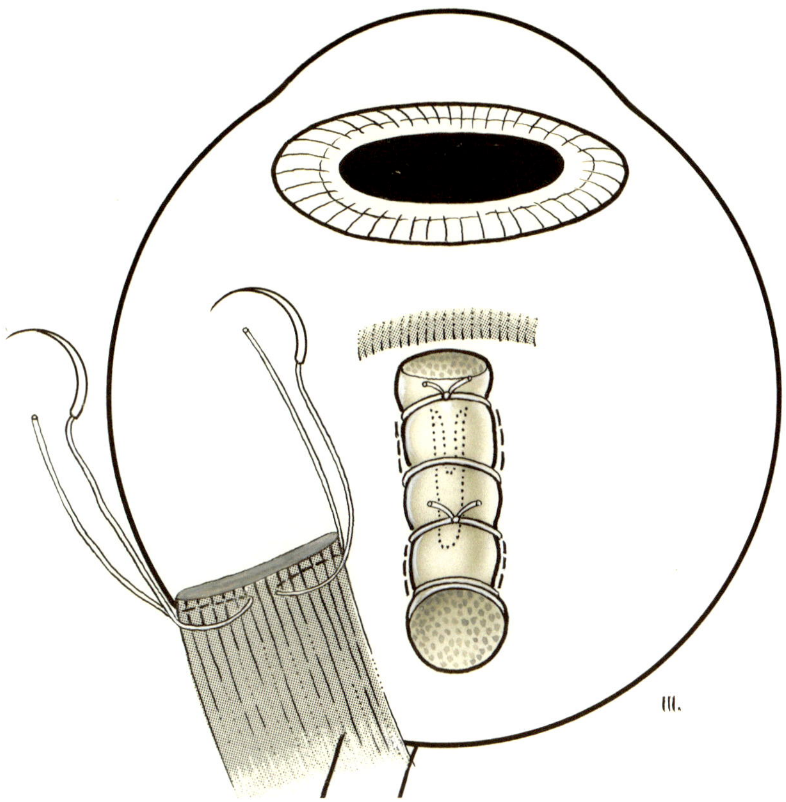

87d

e & f: Alternative type of scleral buckle for repair of retinal hole in the posterior pole of the retina.

g: Sites of retinal fluid drainage in anterior sclera at 7:00 and 11:00 meridians.

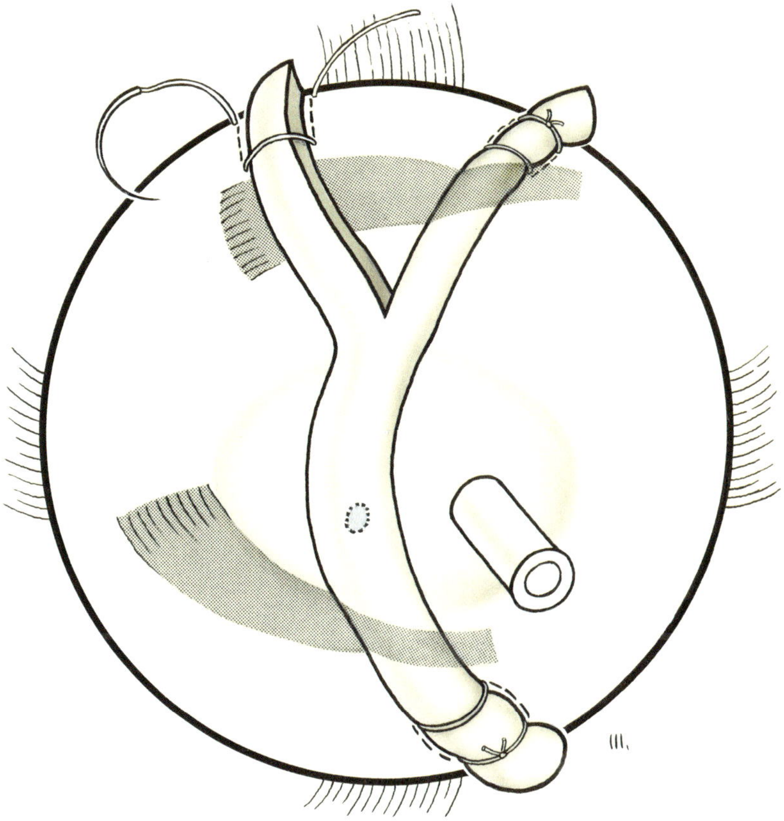

87e

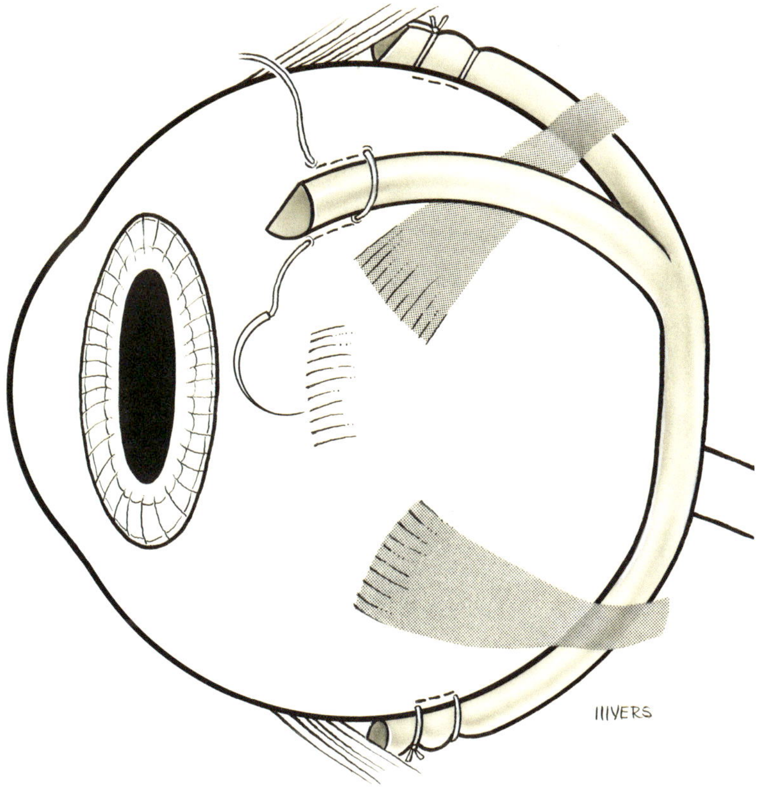

87f

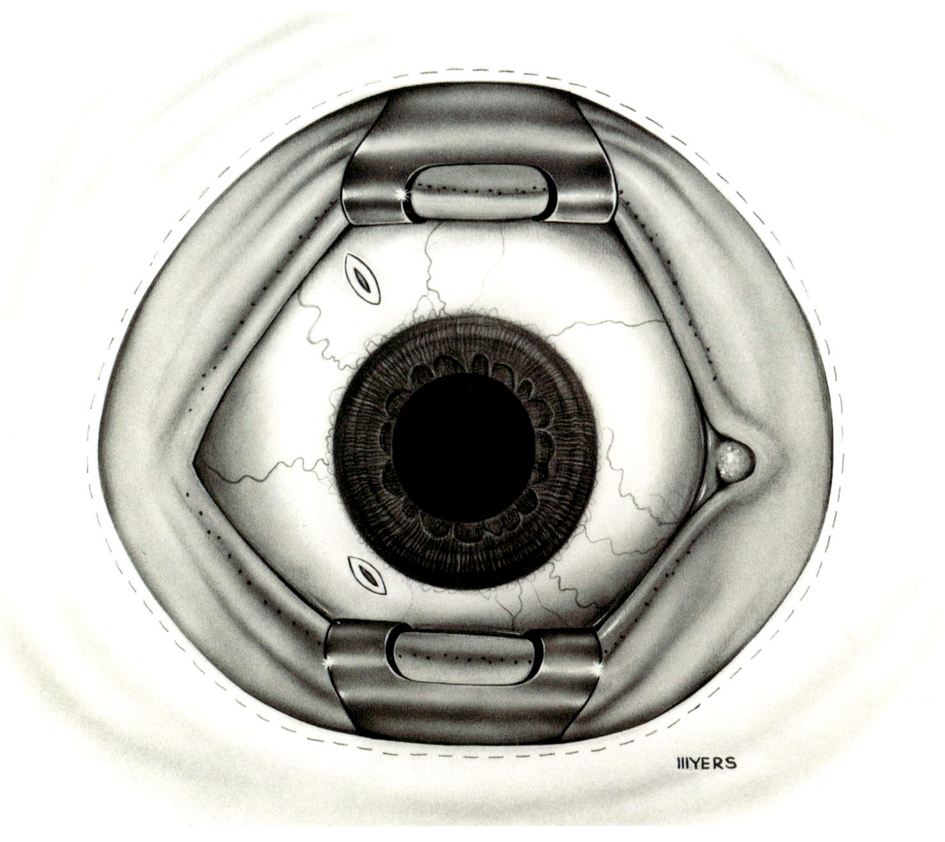

87g

PLATE 88a–q

Photocoagulation to Prevent Reoperation After Scleral Buckling Operations

These seventeen grayscale illustrations were developed to illustrate photocoagulation techniques using the Carl Zeiss photocoagulator. Fourteen illustrations were used in a report by Curtin, Norton and Gass in 1966 at the seventy-first annual meeting of the American Academy of Ophthalmology and Otolaryngology in Chicago, Illinois, USA then published in the Transactions of the American Academy of Ophthalmology and Otolaryngology in 1967 (Curtin VTC, Norton EWD, Gass JDM. Photocoagulation: Its use in the prevention of reoperation after scleral buckling operations. Trans Am Acad Ophthalmol Otolaryngol 1967; 71:432-441).

a–d:

Case 1 illustrates a retinal detachment (a), an anterior route detachment after initial repair by the scleral buckling procedure (b), treatment by photocoagulation (white dots) (c), with attached retina three years later with all subretinal fluid eliminated (d).

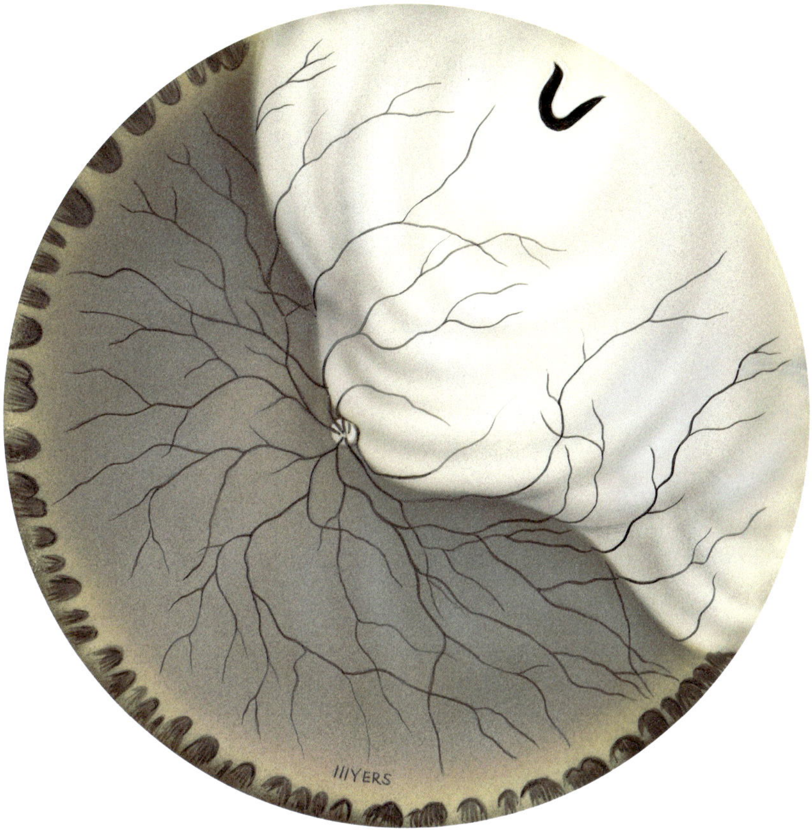

88a

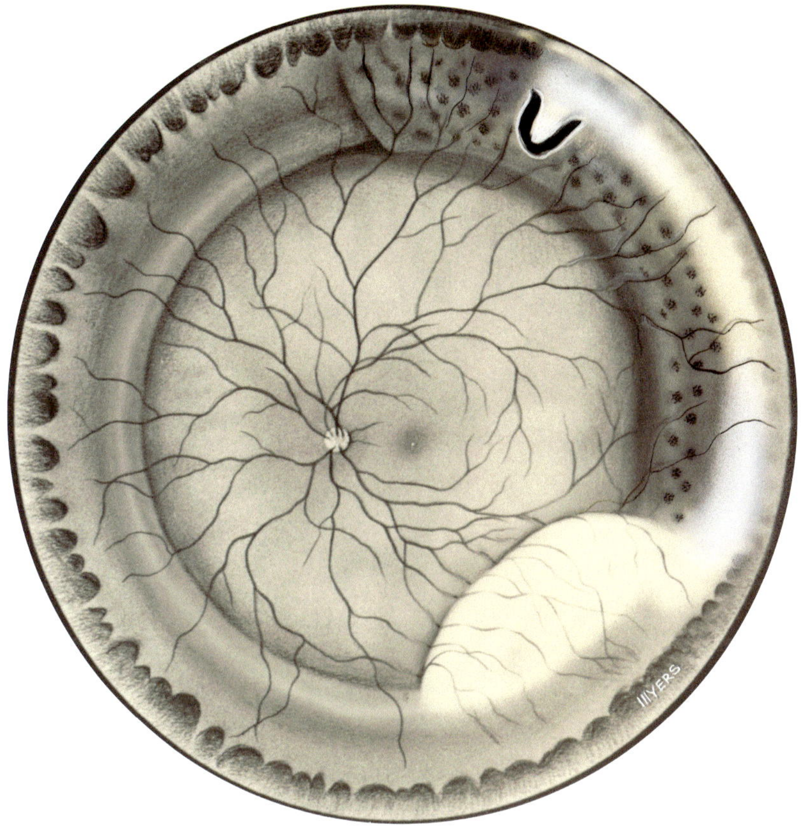

88b

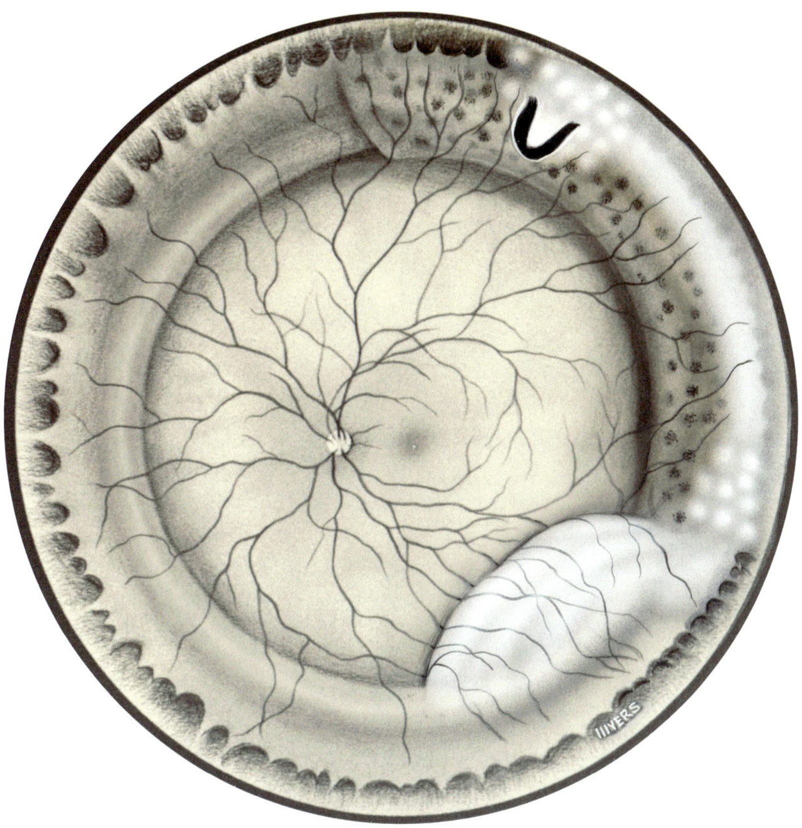

88c

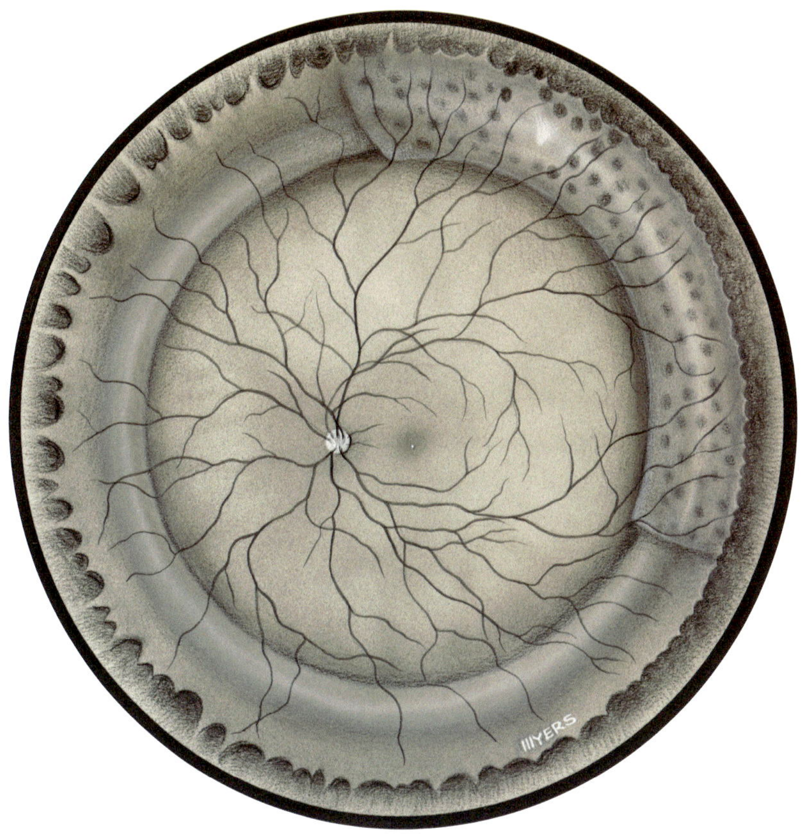

88d

Photocoagulation to Prevent Reoperation After Scleral Buckling Operations

e–h:

Case 2 demonstrates residual subretinal fluid following retinal surgery with a posterior detachment (e), extension of subretinal fluid after three retinal detachment operations (f), treatment by photocoagulation with re-accumulation of fluid (g), the attached retina four years after photocoagulation (h).

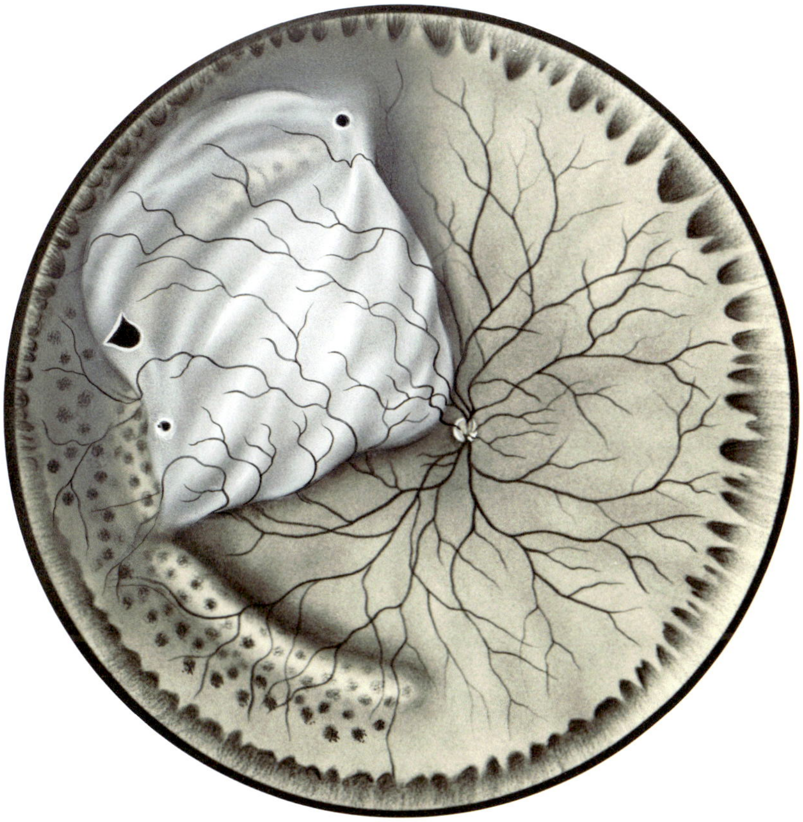
88e

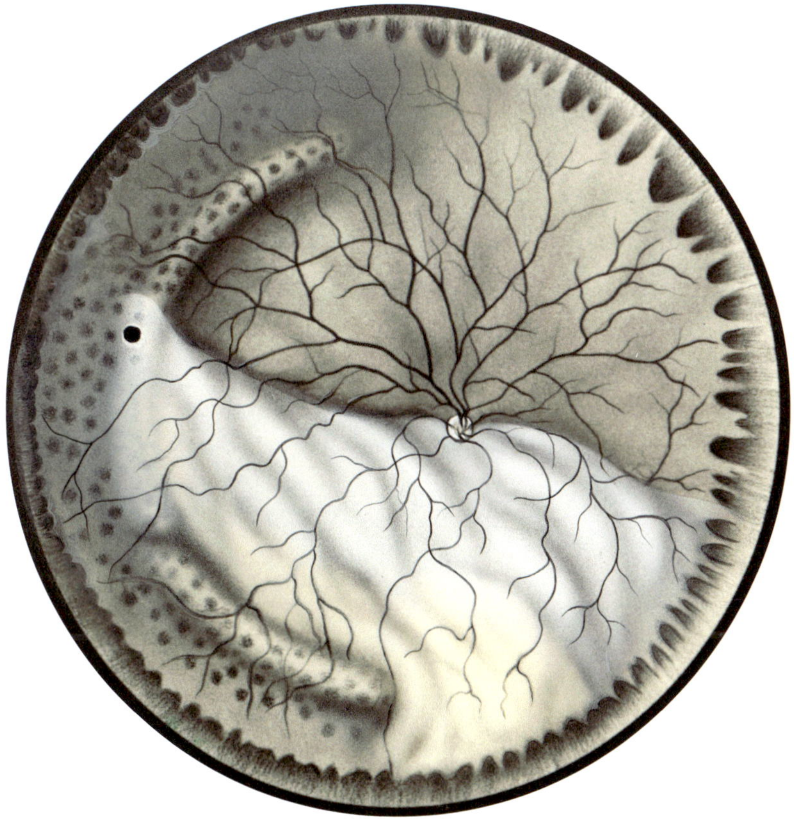
88f

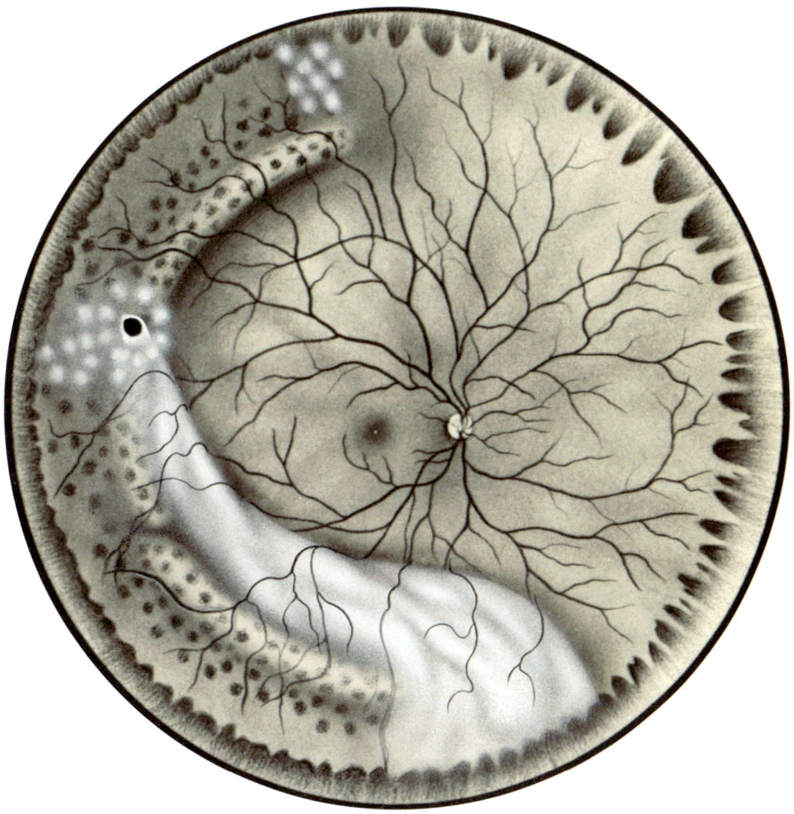
88g

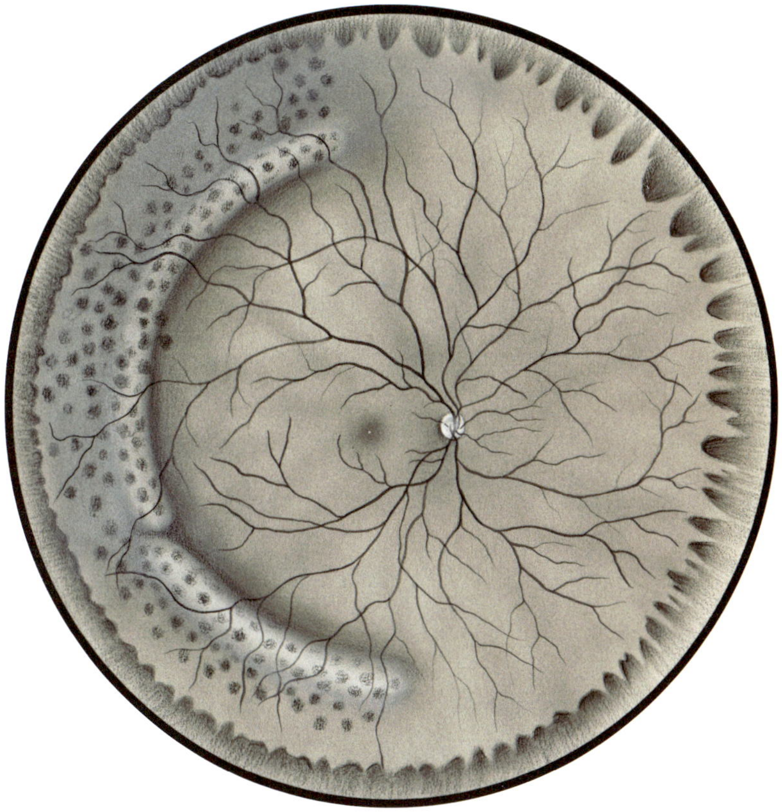
88h

Photocoagulation to Prevent Reoperation After Scleral Buckling Operations

i–l:

Residual subretinal fluid following retinal detachment surgery with retinal elevation anterior to the buckle (i), treatment with localized photocoagulation (j), followed by further photocoagulation (k), appearance of the fundus four years later (l).

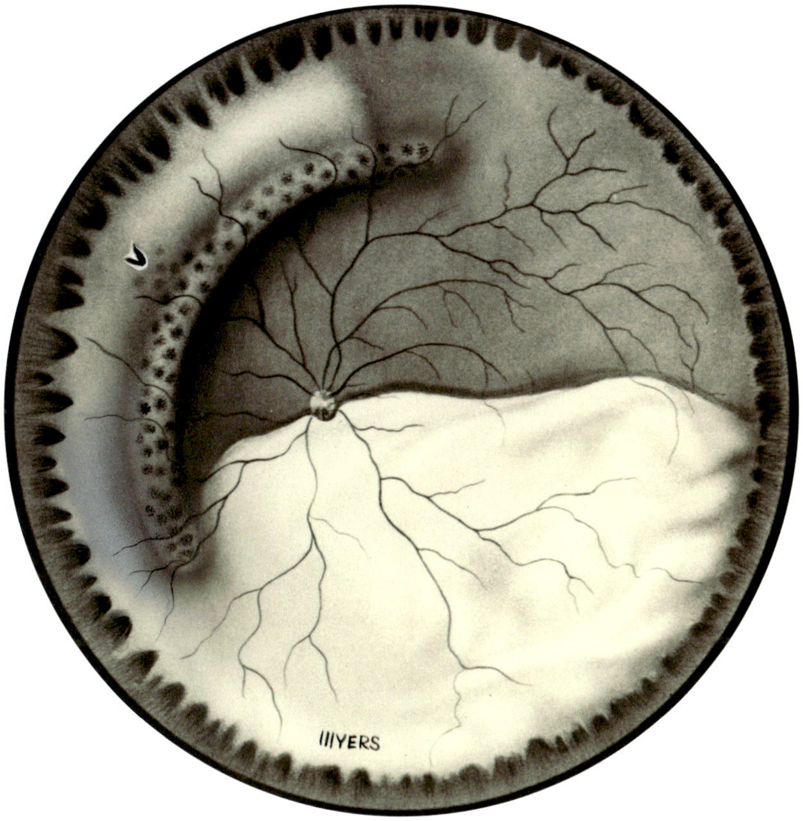

88i

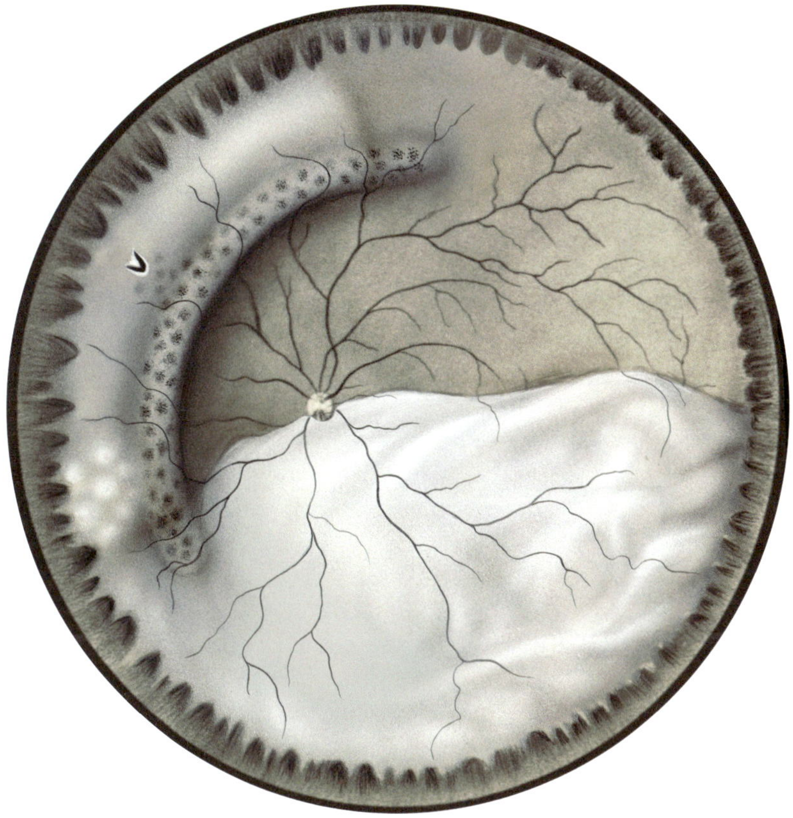

88j

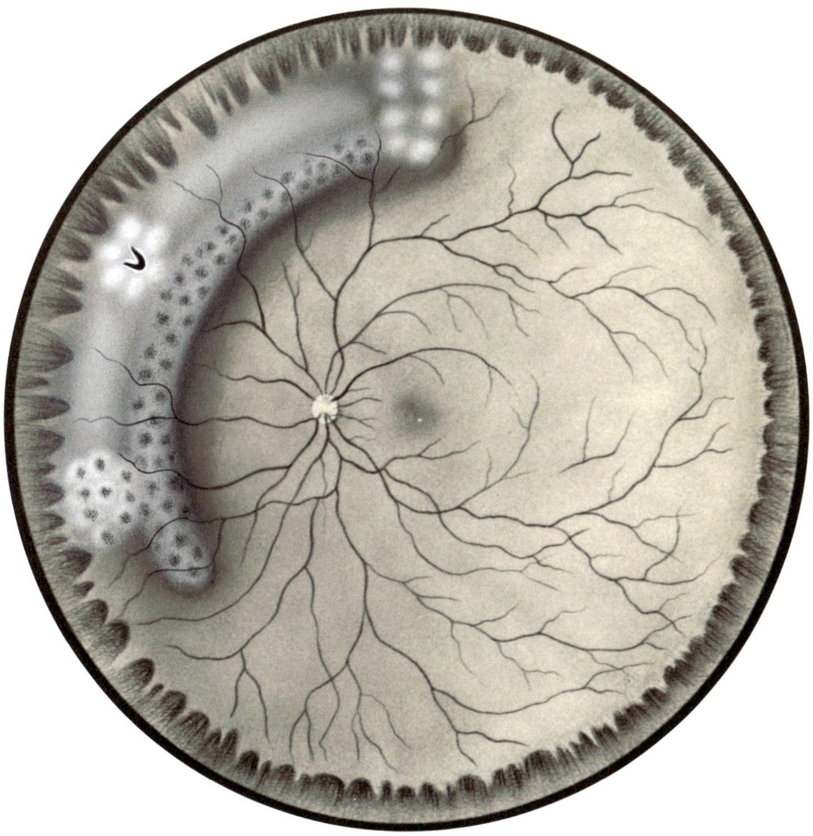

88k

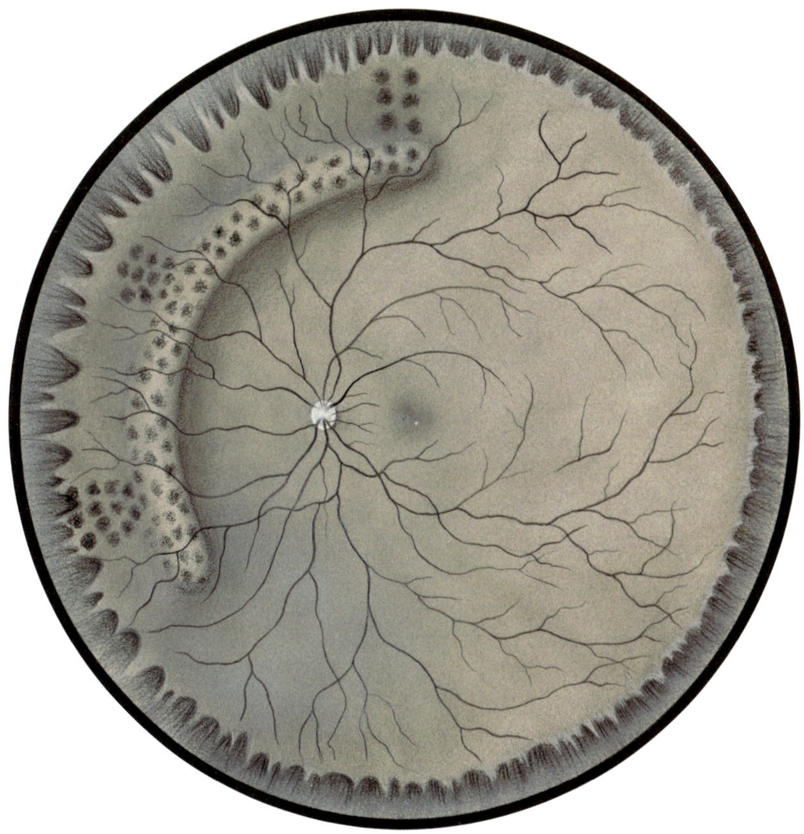

88l

Photocoagulation to Prevent Reoperation After Scleral Buckling Operations

m–p:

Further examples of failed retinal detachment repair which required treatment by photocoagulation.

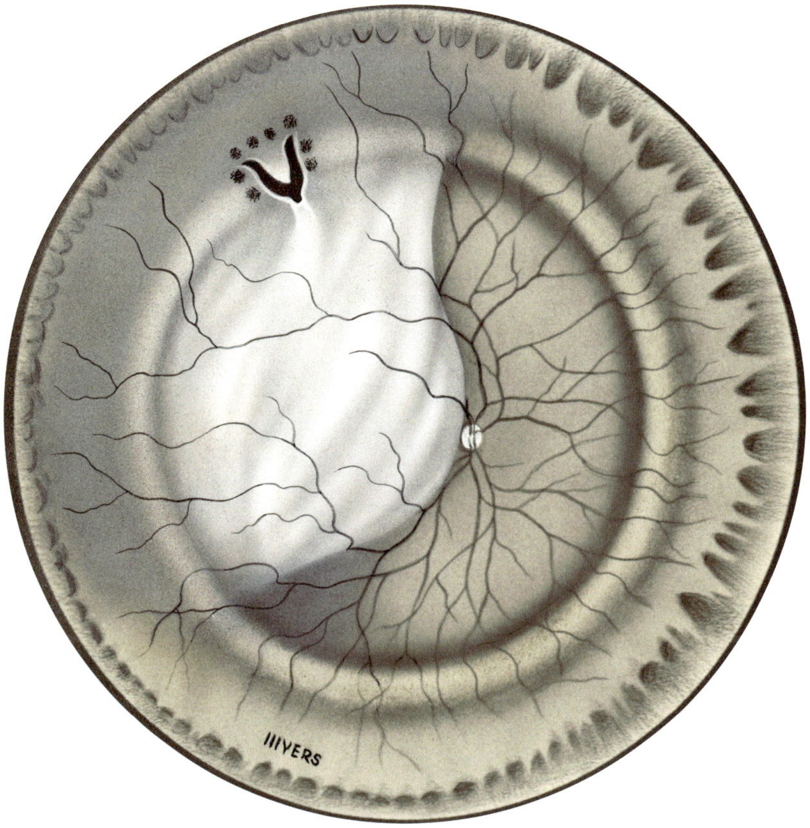

88m

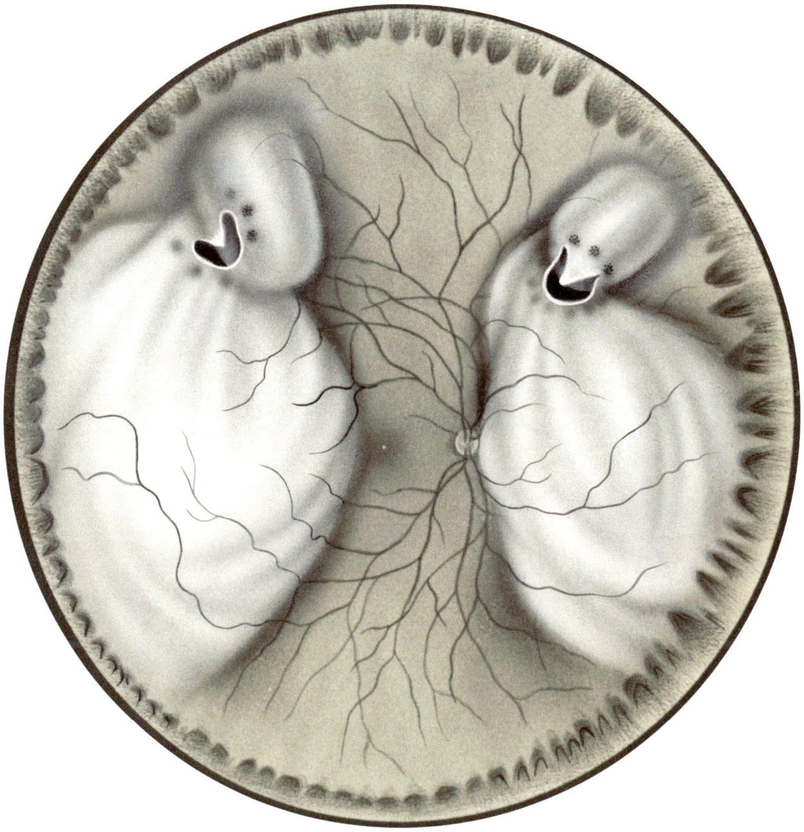

88n

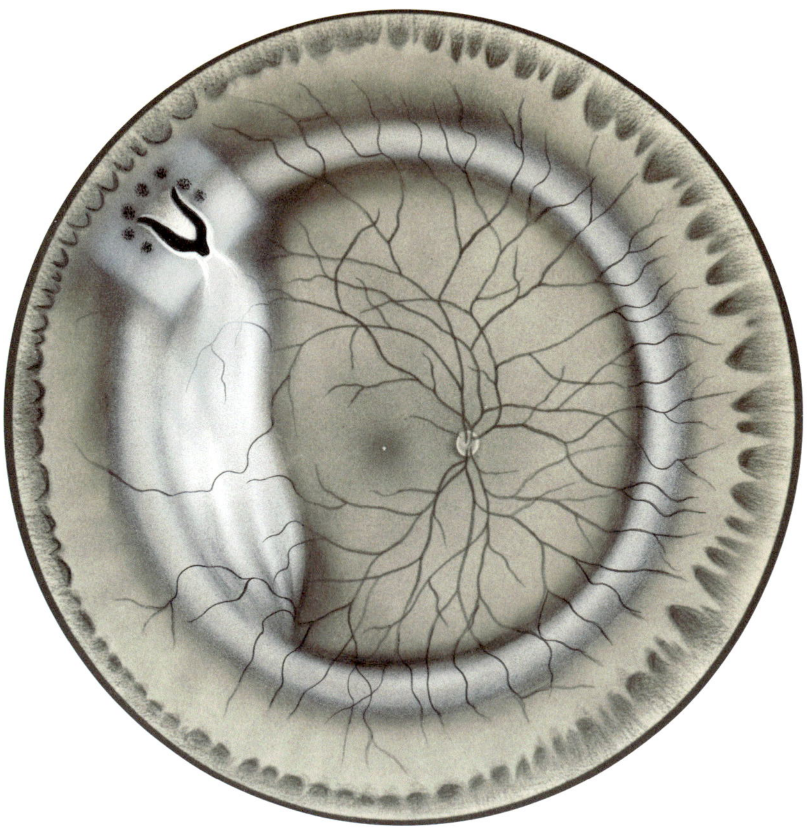

88o

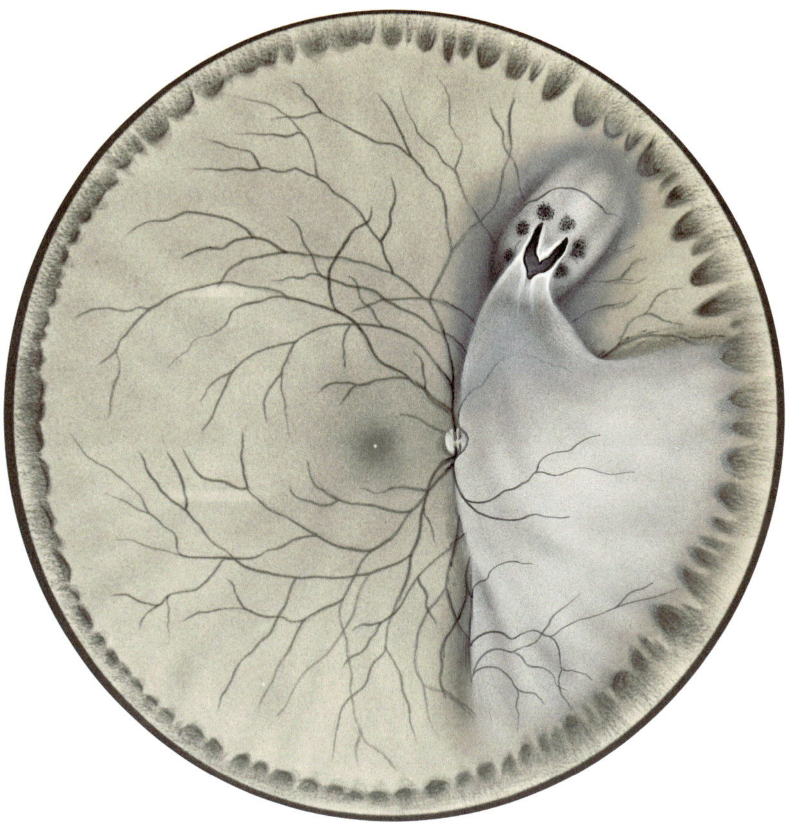

88p

Photocoagulation to Prevent Reoperation After Scleral Buckling Operations

q: This grayscale painting of the fundus was developed as a base illustration, photographed in 8 × 10 inch size, then covered with acetate. Mr. Myers then painted alternative illustrations on and over the acetate to complete the figures in Plate 88.

PLATE 89

Fundus Fluorescein Angiography

This painting is a color schematic depicting the basic optics of intravenous fluorescein angiography. A blue excitation filter is used to illuminate the retina right after the patient has had fluorescein sodium dye infused via the antecubital vein seconds earlier. The circulating dye is excited by the blue light (wavelength 465 nm to 490 nm) from the camera's flash and subsequently fluoresces yellow light (wavelength 525 nm) back to the observer. The fundus camera is equipped with a blue excitation filter and yellow band-pass filter, the latter only allowing yellow light to reach the film of the camera.

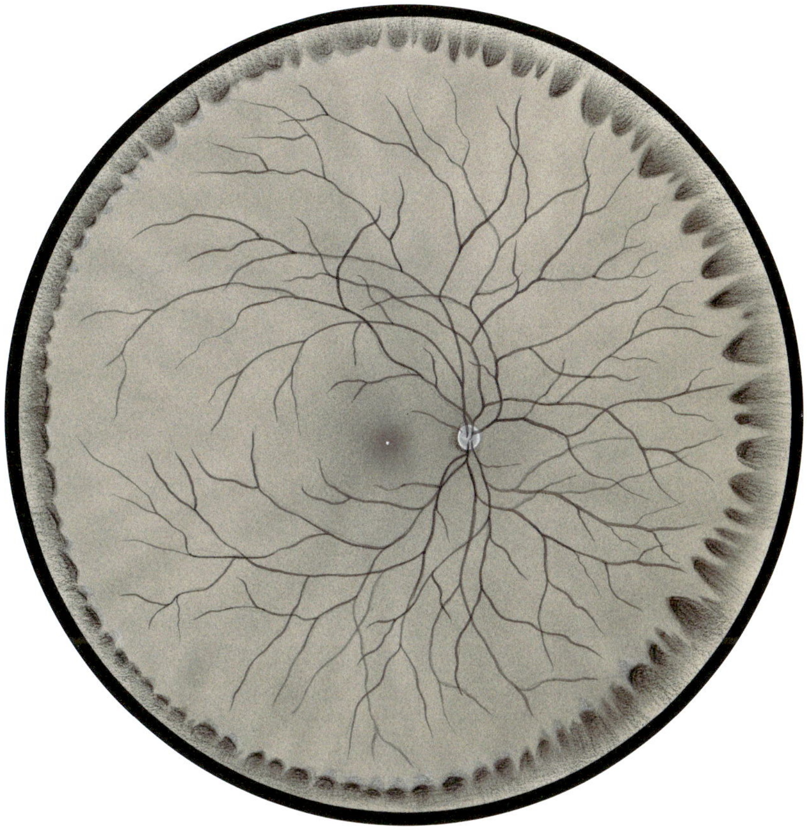

88q

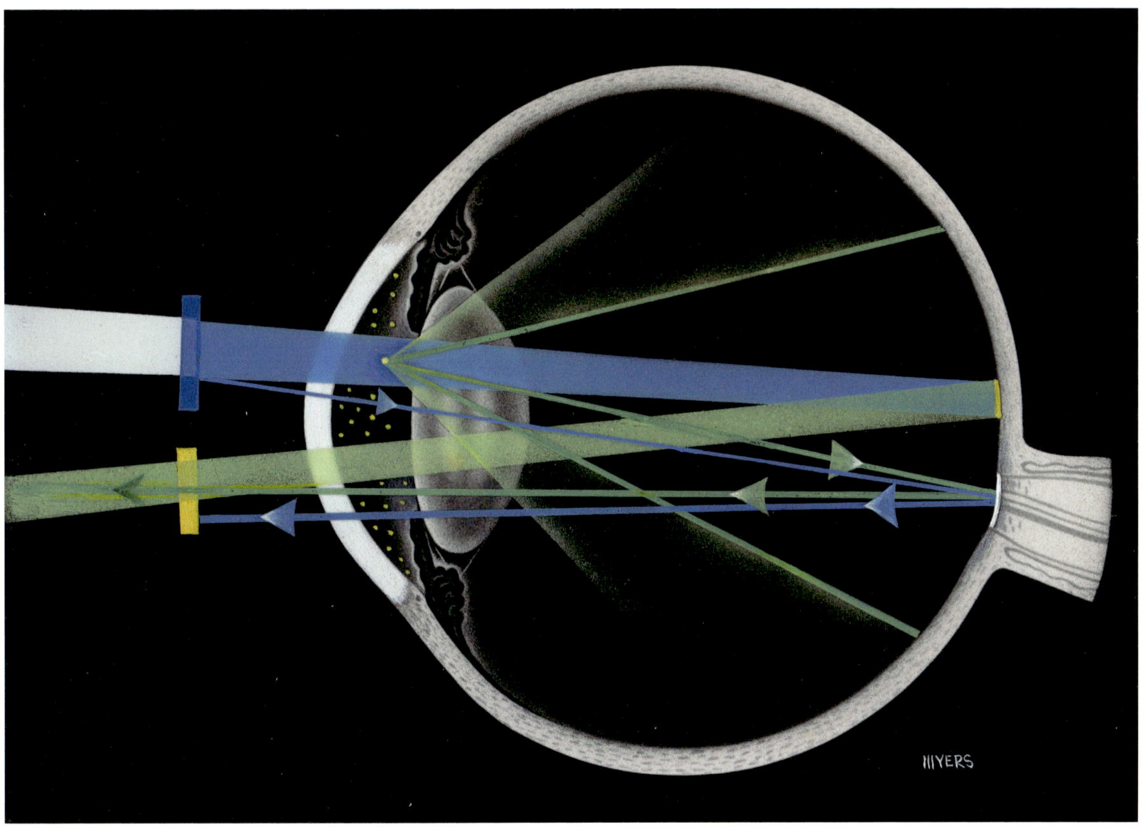

89